GETTING READY TO BE A MOTHER

CHAPTER I
GETTING READY TO BE A MOTHER

How does it seem to you—the coming of a baby?

Does it seem the most amazing of miracles, so stirring in its beauty and mystery that you are eager to make ready and prepare for it fitly?

Or have you, perhaps, come to share the general feeling that motherhood is a natural state which one accepts when it comes, but need not prepare for?

This attitude seems to go back to a very old and deeply rooted conviction that, as women always have had babies and have had them through the working of one of Nature's laws that has been operating over and over throughout the ages, they doubtless will continue to have them in the same old way, and the entire matter may well be left to take care of itself. As to the baby, when he comes, one may expect that the ability to care for him will come too.

Because of this reasoning, or lack of it, it has been a fairly general custom for the woman who expected a baby to seek her doctor's aid only when she went into labor, or shortly beforehand, and to give no thought to the care of her baby until he was born. All too often the mother has died, because of this tardy care, been injured or become an invalid, while equally sad things have happened to the baby—and needlessly so.

But now, happily, a great change is taking place in the realm of mothers and babies. We still realize, of course, that childbearing is a natural function, but we know that conditions must be made favorable for the smooth working of this natural law if all is to be well; that for the sake of both mother and baby it is of urgent importance to give thought and care to the baby during the nine months before he is born.

There is little doubt that the most critical period in one's life is the first ten months—the nine months before birth and the first month afterward—and that the care which is given during these months influences one's physical state, for good or ill, throughout all the rest of life. In the light of this knowledge, women are more and more generally seeking and being given "prenatal care," which is care before the baby is born, together with advice and instructions which fit them to assume motherhood safely and successfully.

Ideal prenatal care would really begin during the expectant mother's own infancy, for the chances of a normal pregnancy, labor and lying-in period are greatly increased by good care during the early years of life. But for the time being we shall have to content ourselves with an effort to extend, as widely as possible, the care that is now known to be beneficial for expectant mothers from the beginning of pregnancy.

This prenatal care is undertaken in much the same spirit in which one makes a garden, for example. We know, of course, that plants which are neglected sometimes grow and blossom satisfactorily, though one would not think of depending upon them to do so. But we have learned that plants that are given the care and protection that they need are almost certain to flourish and bloom after the manner of their kind.

Experience teaches, however, that this care must be regular and sustained and always given for the twofold purpose of preserving the plants from injury as well as nourishing them. Accordingly we put them in good soil, to begin with, and then give water, sunshine or shade, according to their respective needs, and we take care to protect them from the destructive effects of harmful insects, blights, weeds or anything which may be unfavorable to their healthy progress. We do not close our eyes to the fact that these harmful conditions are possible. Instead, we are anxious to find out all about them—what causes them and how to recognize them—in order that we may prevent or remove them before they do serious damage.

Many women, nowadays, are taking just that kind of attitude toward motherhood. They begin by consulting a doctor as soon as they know that they are pregnant, because they appreciate the importance of doing so. They study eagerly the questions relating to motherhood; the structure and workings of those parts of their own bodies which are concerned with the baby's creation; how he evolves within them; what he needs during those nine months of development; what practices, what conditions are bad for the baby and themselves; what they can do to avoid or correct these and how they can help to make things go smoothly.

The women who face the facts of motherhood in this way generally go through the entire adventure normally and successfully, as Nature intended they should. More than this, those women who place themselves under a doctor's care from the beginning of, or early in, pregnancy, are greatly reassured to find out how much can be done to safeguard them, and they do not have that fear of the approaching birth which is suffered by so many women who do not know nor understand what is going on.

The results of the painstaking work and study which have been carried on to increase the comfort and safety of mothers and babies have made it possible for the doctors to plan something of a routine which they find advisable for their patients to adopt. To begin with, it is quite plain that the first need of every expectant mother is examination and measurement, early in pregnancy, by a good physician. The information thus obtained helps the doctor to foretell the kind of labor that his patient is likely to have, and by planning for it ahead of time he is often able to save her much harm and suffering. An early examination also enables the doctor to discover and correct any slight trouble which may exist at that time and which might grow worse if not treated, and to advise his patient about the general care which he wishes her to take of herself throughout pregnancy. In regard to this care, doctors are generally agreed that the average woman needs to do little more than observe the ordinary rules of personal hygiene, which as a matter of fact, should be followed by all of us; that is, she should live a simple, regular life as to diet, fresh air, exercise, rest, sleep, diversions, etc. This all sounds simple enough and as a matter of course, but it is usually overlooked in spite of being of the most urgent importance to both mother and baby.

This advice varies in little things, here and there, among different doctors, but in the main it is about the same the world over, where thought is being given to the care of expectant mothers. For no matter where they are or what their status, their needs in general are the same. They need a doctor's supervision and they need to practice the principles of personal hygiene.

Accordingly, in addition to making an early examination and giving instructions about the regulation of her daily life, the doctor usually wants to see his patient and make certain observations every little while during pregnancy, just to make sure that everything is going as it should and to be in a position to discover the earliest and slightest symptoms of complications.

In the old days there were certain complications associated with childbirth which the doctors did not know how to prevent and sometimes could not cure—complications which were bad for both mother and baby. But now they know a great deal about both preventing and curing even the most serious of these complications. They have discovered, for one thing, that many conditions which give serious trouble during labor, or soon afterwards, actually have their beginnings during pregnancy, and sometimes very early.

Quite evidently, then, it means a great deal to the expectant mother to have the doctor discover and treat these complications before they have had time to become serious. But he can give early treatment only if he knows about the symptoms of the trouble when they first appear. Some of these symptoms may be detected by the expectant mother herself after they have been explained to her, but some of them can be discovered only by a doctor or a nurse. That is why it is important for the doctor to see his patient at frequent intervals during pregnancy; about once a month during the first half and every two weeks afterwards.

He sees her for much the same reasons that the housewife looks over the contents of her darning basket—not once and for all time, but regularly, once a week, over and over and over. She searches each time not for holes alone, but for thin places, too; an occasional broken thread or the beginning of a "run," knowing how much trouble she will save herself, later on, by promptly repairing the smallest break or evidence of wear. She knows quite well that there are no more holes because she looks for them, than there are if she does not, and that failure to look for them will not keep the holes from being there nor from growing larger. No more does the expectant mother develop a complication because she is examined, nor does an existing condition cease to exist because she is not examined; and yet some women still take just that illogical attitude toward examinations and supervision during pregnancy.

One factor which keeps some expectant mothers from seeking medical care is the well-meaning but dangerous counsel so freely offered by older women who claim fitness to advise by virtue of having had several children of their own. Their lack of success, as evidenced by miscarriages, stillbirths, children dying in early infancy, as well as injuries and disabilities of their own, is usually overlooked as they press their superstitions and remedies upon the inexperienced and bewildered younger woman. When disaster follows, as it so often does, it is very likely to be ascribed to the will of God, and the mother's needless sacrifice does not even serve as a warning to others who are in line for the same kind of advice.

Another obstacle to adequate prenatal care is sometimes found in the husband who considers it entirely reasonable to secure expert advice upon the subject of cattle-raising, let us say, or the care and running of his automobile or about his investments, but who has a conviction that it is normal and natural for women to have children without making what he considers a fuss about it. He may cherish, too, a suspicion that it is not altogether good for his wife to be thinking too much about her condition. His mother never began bothering until the baby came.

On the other hand, many husbands show the tenderest solicitude for their wives throughout pregnancy and would be only too eager to have them enjoy all the benefits of prenatal care, if they only knew and understood about it. The expectant mother will be wise, therefore, if she undertakes to convince her husband, if need be, that her occupation of bearing and rearing children merits quite the same thoughtful attention as his work, to which he devotes his best powers.

How easy and worth while this may be was demonstrated a couple of years ago at a county fair which was attended by a very intelligent farmer and his wife. The farmer was interested in hog-raising and both he and his wife accepted without question the fact that success in this enterprise could be achieved only through serious study and the most painstaking care. But as to childbearing, if they thought of it at all, they looked upon it as simply one of those natural functions which always had and doubtless always would take care of itself.

When this couple reached the fair the farmer entered one of his fine animals in a prize-winning contest and as there was a baby contest, too, the wife entered their little son. In due time the judges inspected the various contestants and it was found that point by point the farmer's hog measured up to all of the standards of perfection for his kind and easily won the first prize. Not so with the baby; point by point he fell below even a moderate average of what a baby should be and was outranked by many of his more robust infant competitors.

As various admirers discussed hog-raising with the farmer, it became quite evident that he had carefully studied the question and had applied to his occupation the most approved methods of which he could learn. But when the doctors and nurses at the baby contest talked with the crestfallen mother about her baby, who had seemed right enough to her, they found that she knew little or nothing of the business of being a mother; that it had never occurred to her nor to her husband that she might profit by care and instruction about herself and her baby both before and after he was born. As might be expected, she had been unable to nurse him and on the whole he proved to be a pretty poor specimen of a baby, with a dismal outlook as to health.

Since the mother was then in an early stage of another pregnancy, the doctor talked it all over with her and her husband. He convinced them that such thoughtful and painstaking care as they had devoted successfully to hog-raising were equally effective when applied to baby-raising. As a result, the expectant mother, with her husband's whole-hearted approval, placed herself under the care and supervision which she found were available through a prenatal clinic in her vicinity.

The happy sequel to that story is that when another fair was held, a year later, the farmer entered another one of his hogs and the wife her new baby, and that this baby held his own with the hog by taking a prize, too.

So sincerely do doctors now believe in the urgency of having all maternity patients under supervision and care during the nine months before the baby comes and the first several weeks afterwards, that they not only care for those women who come to their offices, but also give of their knowledge and skill to organizations engaged in prenatal and maternity work. These organizations may be visiting nurse associations, prenatal clinics, health centers or dispensaries. As the doctors are assisted by nursing staffs they are able to offer protection, through these channels, to a very large number of mothers and babies.

Among the women who are cared for by such organizations, or by doctors in their private practice, there is an enormous reduction in the occurrence of convulsions, for example, abortions, miscarriages, stillbirths, infections (childbed fever), and prolonged and difficult labors. Or, to put it the other way round, good care started during early pregnancy and continued throughout labor and the lying-in period gives both mother and baby enormously increased chances to live and enjoy good health. One reason why the baby is so much better off is that good care practically always enables his mother to nurse him, for, except in extremely rare cases when there is a definite physical disability, as tuberculosis for example, every mother can nurse her baby if she really wants to and if she, the doctor and nurse bend all their energies to accomplish this happy end. A baby who is not breast-fed is defrauded of a protection which is rightfully his, and usually because someone has failed to do all in his or her power.

Organizations which include doctors and nurses who can give skilled care to maternity patients are increasing in scope and number throughout cities, towns and rural districts in all parts of the country. This makes us hope that before long good care during pregnancy, childbirth and young motherhood will be available to every woman in the land. But quite as earnestly do we also hope that every woman in the land who is looking forward to motherhood will seek this care. Certain it is that the expectant mother who does seek care, whether from a doctor in his office or through a prenatal clinic, is approaching her motherhood in the only way that is safe for herself and her baby. She should realize, however, that although the doctors can accomplish a great deal through examinations and advice, they can give the full benefits of their skill only to those women who do their part by following instructions faithfully, week after week, throughout nine months. The doctor cannot live his patient's life for her; he can plan and advise her ever so wisely, but this counts for very little unless she lives as he directs.

The young woman who sees her motherhood as a coveted privilege, crowded with happy possibilities, who is willing to bear its inconveniences and take the necessary precautions to insure a satisfactory outcome, is very likely to go through her experience in good health and buoyant spirits. And in the end she will have not only the ecstasy of possessing a beautiful, well baby who has every prospect of continuing so, but as the years pass she will have the satisfaction of knowing that she is a better, more helpful, more companionable mother because of being in good health herself.

That is the point of good maternity care—future well-being as well as immediate safety for both mother and baby—and it rests with each woman to decide for herself if she is to have such care.

CHAPTER II
SIGNS THAT A BABY IS COMING

The woman who wants a baby and is in a position to have one is usually eager to know how she can tell when a baby is coming. She wants to know because the baby's coming means so much to her and also in order that she may know when to consult a doctor.

I am sorry to have to admit, at the outset, that making this important discovery is far from being a simple matter. One would suppose, after all these ages, during which countless babies have been born and countless pregnancies have been observed by doctors and others, that there would be some known way of finding out definitely, at an early date, whether or not a baby was coming. But strangely enough, there is no positive evidence of the baby's existence within his mother's body until eighteen or twenty weeks after his life there has begun.

On the other hand, so many symptoms of pregnancy are known to women, the world over, that very often an expectant mother is correct when she suspects at an early date that she is pregnant, particularly if she has already had a child. But as the well-known symptoms are much like those of various conditions other than pregnancy, even experienced mothers sometimes believe themselves pregnant when they are not. The reverse is true also, for we occasionally hear of a woman who fails to recognize the meaning of the changes which she notices in herself, and is unaware of being pregnant up to the very time of going into labor.

And so we find that there are some signs of pregnancy which are only *possible*, since they may be caused by some other conditions; others which may be accepted as *probable*, and a few signs which are *positive* because they are never due to any cause but pregnancy.

The **possible** signs can all be detected by the expectant mother, herself, and may be described as follows:

1. **Stopping of Menstruation.** This is usually the first symptom noticed. Although it is possible for the periods to be stopped by any one of several other causes, the missing of two successive periods, after intercourse, is a strong indication of pregnancy in a healthy woman of the childbearing age, whose menses have been regular.

2. **Changes in the Breasts.** These, also, occur early. The breasts usually increase in size and firmness, and many women complain of throbbing, tingling or pricking sensations and a feeling of tightness and fullness. The breasts may be so tender that even slight pressure is painful. The nipples become larger and more prominent; they and the colored circle of skin around them grow darker, while the veins and the glands that feel like little lumps under the skin become more noticeable. If, in addition to these symptoms, it is possible for a woman who has not had children to squeeze from her nipples a pale yellowish fluid, called colostrum, she may feel almost certain that she is pregnant. But it must be remembered that these symptoms, also, may be due to causes other than pregnancy; that even milk in the breasts may be present in a woman who has borne children, for months, or possibly years, after the birth of her last baby.

3. "**Morning sickness**," as the name suggests, is nausea, sometimes accompanied by vomiting, from which many expectant mothers suffer the first thing in the morning. This varies from a little nausea, when first raising her head, to repeated attacks of vomiting during the day and even during the night. As a rule, however, the discomfort is experienced during the early part of the day only. Morning sickness may set in immediately after conception, but begins about the sixth week, as a rule, and lasts until the third or fourth month. It occurs in about half of all pregnancies and is particularly common among women who are pregnant for the first time. On the other hand, one must not forget that many non-pregnant women suffer from nausea in the morning; many women go through pregnancy without any such disturbance, while others are entirely comfortable in the morning but nauseated during the latter part of the day.

4. **Frequent Urination.** There is usually a desire to pass urine frequently during the first three or four months of pregnancy, after which the tendency disappears, but returns during the later months. The desire may be due in

part to nervousness, but is largely caused by pressure made upon the bladder by the growing baby, and not by kidney trouble, as is sometimes believed. For pressure on the outside of the bladder gives much the same sensation as is experienced when the bladder is full of urine. After the baby grows to such a size that he pushes up into the abdomen (we shall describe this later), he does not press upon the bladder and therefore ceases to create a desire to urinate until the last month or six weeks before he is born when he sinks back into the pelvis.

5. **Increased discoloration** of the colored parts of the skin is another early symptom of pregnancy. In addition to the deepened tint of the nipples and the circles around them, a dark streak appears upon the lower part of the abdomen, extending upward toward the umbilicus, or navel. There are also the yellowish, irregularly shaped blotches which sometimes appear upon the face and neck; dark circles under the eyes and pinkish or bluish streaks on the abdomen.

6. "**Quickening**" is the name which is commonly given to the mother's first feeling of the baby's movements. It occurs about the eighteenth or twentieth week, and is regarded by some doctors as a positive sign of pregnancy and by others as merely a possible sign. The sensation is compared to a very slight quivering, or tapping, or to the fluttering of the wings of a bird as it is held in one's hand. Beginning very gently, these movements grow more vigorous, as time goes on, until they become very troublesome toward the latter part of pregnancy, amounting then to sharp kicks and blows. Women who have had children can usually distinguish between quickening and the somewhat similar sensation caused by the movement of gas in the intestines; but a woman pregnant for the first time may be deceived.

There are many other possible symptoms of pregnancy, but their value is very uncertain and as we have seen, even the ones described above are not entirely dependable. But if you have missed two periods; if your breasts have grown larger and firmer; if your nipples are stiffer and more prominent and you can squeeze colostrum from them, you may be reasonably certain that a baby is coming.

The **probable signs** of pregnancy are more apparent to the doctor than to the expectant mother, but there are two which you may easily detect:

1. **Enlargement of the abdomen**, which is a very important sign, may be noticed about the third month. At this stage a rounded mass may be felt in the abdomen which steadily increases in size as the weeks and months slip by. Rapid enlargement of the abdomen in a woman of childbearing age may be taken as fair, but not positive, evidence that she is carrying a baby. However, complete reliance cannot be placed in this sign, since it is possible for the abdomen to be enlarged by a tumor, by dropsy, or by fat.

2. **Painless contractions of the uterus** (or womb, within which the baby lies) begin during the early weeks of pregnancy and occur at intervals of five or ten minutes throughout the entire period. The expectant mother may not be conscious of these contractions during the early months, but later she can detect them by placing her hand upon her abdomen and feeling the uterus, beneath it, grow first hard and then soft, as it contracts and relaxes. But the probable signs of pregnancy, like the possible symptoms, may occur in women who are not pregnant, and accordingly the appearance of any one of them alone, is not of great significance.

The **positive signs** of pregnancy, of which there are three, are not apparent until the eighteenth or twentieth week. They relate to the baby, but with one exception they cannot be detected by the expectant mother. However, they are of such moment that you will be interested to know what they are.

1. **Hearing and counting the baby's heart beat** is unmistakable evidence of the baby's existence. The doctor sometimes hears this by resting his ear upon the mother's abdomen and sometimes by listening through a stethoscope.

2. **Ability to feel the outline of the baby's body** is also a positive sign of pregnancy, if the head, buttocks, back and extremities are unmistakably made out through the mother's abdominal wall.

3. **Feeling the movements of the baby** is accepted as a third positive sign of pregnancy. There is some difference of opinion concerning the value of "quickening," alone, as a positive sign, but if the baby's movements are felt by the doctor, also, through the mother's abdominal wall, or by vaginal examination, there can be no doubt that a baby is there. Feeling these movements some time after the eighteenth or twentieth week, by placing a hand upon the abdomen, is the one positive sign which the expectant mother may detect for herself.

Some Other Changes in the Mother's Body While the Baby Grows. In addition to the signs and symptoms which we have just described, there are a good many other changes which will take place in your own body, in the course of the baby's development, and you will want to learn about some of them in order that you may know what to expect.

The abdomen. Of course, the steady enlargement of the abdomen and the alteration in its shape, as pregnancy advances, is the change that you will be most conscious of. As the abdomen grows larger, the skin which covers it is stretched more and more tightly with the result that the tissues just under the surface sometimes give way, or split and form pale pink or bluish streaks. These streaks, which are called *striæ*, grow white and glistening after the baby is born, so that the abdomen of an expectant mother who has had children, will show silvery streaks from earlier pregnancies and also the bluish ones recently formed. These streaks are of no consequence and I mention them simply because you are almost certain to notice them and may wonder what they are. They may appear upon the hips, thighs and breasts as well as upon the abdomen, if the skin over these parts is greatly stretched.

The umbilicus (navel) is deeply indented during about the first three months of pregnancy, but afterwards the pit steadily grows shallower and by the seventh month, it is level with the surface of the abdomen. After this time the navel may protrude, in which state it is described as a "pouting umbilicus."

An increase in the vaginal discharge is another change which you may notice during the latter months of pregnancy.

The changes in the skin consist chiefly of the increased discoloration over various parts of the body, which was mentioned among the possible signs of pregnancy. The degree of this discoloration varies with the complexion of the individual, as blonds may be tinted but slightly more than usual, while the discolored areas on a brunette may become almost black. As the skin glands become more active, there is also an increase in perspiration and sometimes the hair becomes much more luxuriant during pregnancy.

Changes in the digestive tract are the morning sickness already described, and constipation. The latter is suffered by at least one half of all pregnant women and is due chiefly to pressure made upon the intestines by the enlarged uterus, though weakening of the stretched abdominal muscles may be one cause. Constipation is most troublesome during the latter part of pregnancy. There may be, also, heartburn, acid stomach and intestinal indigestion giving rise to gas, diarrhea and cramps. The so-called "cravings" of pregnancy are not so common in real life as they are in rumor, but the expectant mother may show unexpected likes and dislikes for certain dishes, possibly because of her tendency to be nauseated. Her appetite may be very capricious during the early weeks and become almost ravenous later on.

The bones and teeth may grow softer during pregnancy, if the expectant mother does not eat proper food, and as a result we hear of the old beliefs that each baby costs the mother a tooth and that broken bones heal slowly during pregnancy. Both of these occurrences are entirely unnecessary, and may be prevented by eating suitable food, as will be explained in the chapter on nutrition.

The carriage, or mode of walking, is somewhat affected by pregnancy because of the increased size and weight of the abdomen. In an effort, to hold herself erect, the expectant mother throws back her head and shoulders and finally assumes a gait that may be described as a waddle, being particularly noticeable in short women.

You hear a good deal about the **thyroid gland** these days, so you may as well know that it is very often enlarged during pregnancy and thus may form a swelling on the front part of the neck. If you notice it you might tell your doctor but it need not worry you for it will almost certainly return to its normal size after the baby comes.

When to Expect the Baby. Now that you are familiar with the most apparent changes which will take place in your body during pregnancy, you are probably on tiptoe to find out as nearly as possible the date upon which to expect the baby. Unfortunately we cannot foretell the exact date, for the very simple reason that we have no way of knowing just when pregnancy begins. Quite evidently, then, not knowing when it begins we cannot figure out the exact date upon which pregnancy will end in the baby's birth. But we do know that labor usually begins about ten lunar months, or forty weeks, or from 273 to 280 days, after the beginning of the last menstrual period. Thus the approximate date of the baby's arrival may be estimated by counting forward 280 days or backward 85 days from the first day of the last period. Or, what is perhaps simpler and amounts to the same thing, one may add seven days to the first day of the last period and count back three months. For example, if the last period began on June 3, the addition of seven days brings us to June 10, while counting back three months from this, indicates March 10 as the approximate date upon which the baby may be expected.

This is probably as satisfactory as any method of estimation, but at best it is only approximate, being accurate in about one case in twenty. However, it comes within a week of being correct in half the cases; and is within two weeks of the actual date in eighty per cent. of all pregnancies.

Still another method is to count forward twenty or twenty-two weeks from the day upon which you first feel the baby move. This "quickening," as we have seen, usually occurs about the eighteenth or twentieth week, but is so irregular that it is not wholly reliable. The possibility of figuring out the date of the baby's arrival is made still more uncertain by the fact that there is evidently considerable variation in the length of entirely normal pregnancies. Many healthy children are born before ten lunar months have elapsed since the last menstrual period, while more births occur after than on the expected date. The first pregnancy is usually shorter than later ones, and women who are well nourished and well cared for usually have longer pregnancies than those who are not.

Taking it as a whole, the average woman has unusually good health during pregnancy. She may feel some weariness during the first few months and she may lose a little weight, but during the latter part of the period her general health is improved and there is an increase of flesh, not alone in the abdomen, but over the entire body, sometimes amounting to twenty-five or thirty pounds. She loses about fifteen pounds of the increased weight when the baby is born, and still more during the weeks immediately following, when her body returns to about its original condition. But very often the experience of pregnancy is so beneficial that the improved state of health and nutrition which accompany it become permanent.

CHAPTER III
WHERE THE BABY'S LIFE BEGINS

As you plan for the care of your baby during the nine months before he is born, you will want to know something of the place where his life begins; where one tiny cell is so miraculously stimulated and nourished that it finally develops into a beautiful little body. Not only will you find all of this of absorbing interest, but a general idea of the structures and workings of those parts of your body where the baby lives and grows will help you better to understand some of the doctor's precautions and to give yourself intelligent care while your body performs its supreme function.

To begin with, there is the **pelvis**. This is a very irregular, bottomless, bony basin, or curved canal, within which lie the reproductive or *generative organs* to be described presently. The pelvis is really composed of four bones which are entirely separate in early life but firmly welded into one rigid structure in adults. I mention this because many women believe that labor pains are caused by a spreading or opening of these bones, whereas, as we shall see presently, the pains are really due to the strong contractions of the muscles of the uterus (or womb) in which the baby lies, which force the baby down through this inflexible ring. You may see in Fig. [1] how the pelvis is placed in the body, being interposed between the spinal column, which it supports, and the thighs upon which it rests. We can feel two of its prominent points on either side below the waist, as our hips, and we rest upon two other projections while in the sitting position.

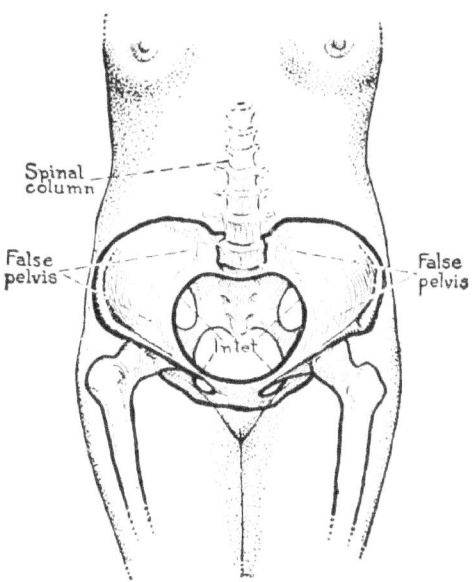

Fig. 1.—Diagram showing the structure of the pelvis and its position in the body, the inlet being heavily outlined.

This bony canal is drawn in, or narrowed about midway in its length so that it is broader above and below than it is in the middle. You are likely to hear the doctors speak of this narrow part as the inlet. I thought you would be interested to know about this for it is largely in order to discover the size and shape of the inlet that the doctor is so anxious to make certain examinations and measurements.

The wide part of the pelvis above the inlet is called the upper, or *false pelvis*, while the smaller cavity below is known as the *true pelvis*. During the early part of pregnancy the baby lies in the true pelvis, but as pregnancy advances and he grows larger, he pushes up through the inlet into the larger pelvis where he remains until he is born. When that time comes he must pass down through the inlet again on his way into the world. If this opening is about the usual size and shape and the baby is of an average size, he will usually pass through with comparatively little trouble. But if the inlet is smaller than normal or of an unusual shape, it may be difficult, or even impossible, for the head of a normal-sized baby to pass through without the doctor's assistance. You can see how important it is, therefore, for the doctor to know beforehand about the size and shape of the pelvic inlet, since it enables him to plan to help with the birth, if necessary, thus saving mother and baby from exhausting themselves in trying to do the impossible.

In the old days many mothers and babies were injured, and sometimes even lost their lives, because doctors did not know about measuring the pelvis and planning ahead of time for a difficult labor. But now they know how to make things easier and safer.

It is worth mentioning here that proper care during infancy and childhood, with proper food, fresh air and exercise, helps to promote normal development of the pelves of little girls, and this in turn tends to make childbirth normal for these children when they grow up and are ready to have babies of their own.

The Generative or Reproductive Organs. The pelvis is an interesting structure but not nearly so interesting as the generative organs which lie within it: the *uterus* (or womb), *tubes* and *ovaries*. These, with the vagina, are often called the *internal genitalia* because they are inside the body. The pelvis practically remains rigid and inactive throughout pregnancy and labor, but the ovaries and the uterus are constantly active and are concerned with an undertaking which is so utterly amazing that it is far beyond our powers of understanding. We can only look on and wonder.

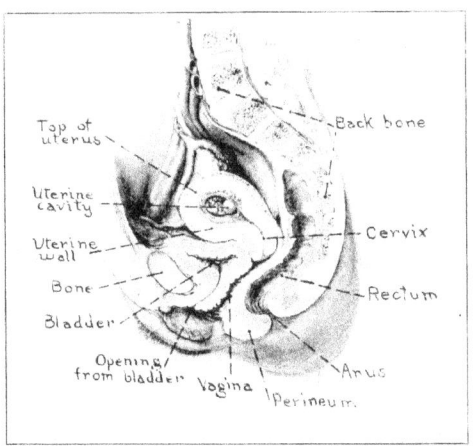

FIG. 2.—Drawing showing the structure and relation of the female generative organs, as viewed from the side. (Drawn by Max Brödel. Used by permission of A. J. Nystrom and Co., Chicago.)

The uterus, or womb, in which the baby develops, is a firm little mass of muscle, which, in its non-pregnant state, is much the shape of a slightly flattened pear, about three inches high, an inch and a quarter wide at its broadest point, three quarters of an inch thick, and weighs about two ounces. We usually speak of the main part of the uterus as the *body*: the round top as the *fundus* and the smaller part of the organ, below, as the neck or cervix. This important little organ is placed about the middle of the true pelvis, with the upper end pointing slightly forward. (See Fig. 2.) It is more or less swung in this position by being attached to ligaments instead of to any fixed part, the ligaments, in turn being attached to the sides of the pelvis. This explains why the uterus may move about, tip forward or backward, and how, by a stretching of the ligaments that hold it, it is able to grow and push upwards as pregnancy advances.

Within the body of the uterus is a flat cavity which is somewhat triangular in shape, with an opening at each of the three corners. The two upper openings lead into the tubes, which will be described in a moment, while a third opening leads down into the cervix, the lower end of the cervix, in turn, protruding into the vagina. The upper and lower ends of the cervix are drawn in as though with a draw string so that they are scarcely more than small round holes. These are called the *internal os* and the *external os*. Fig. 3 gives an idea of how the cavity of the uterus and the cervix would look from the front, with the tubes reaching out from the upper corners of the uterus, and the cervix opening into the vagina. The uterus is lined with a soft mucous lining something like the lining of one's mouth. Bear this in mind, for this lining represents, in part, the soil in which the tiny human seed is planted and through which its roots draw nourishment.

The Fallopian tubes are two little muscular passage ways, about five inches long, which extend from the two upper corners of the uterine cavity toward the sides of the pelvis. The tubes are very small where they arise from the uterus, but gradually grow larger toward their free ends and finally spread out into wide, funnel-shaped openings that lead directly into the abdominal cavity. The tubes, also, are lined with a mucous membrane but of a most surprising kind. Its surface is covered with tiny hair-like projections which make it something like a brush with very soft, moist bristles. These little hairs are in constant motion, waving and sweeping along in much the same way that a field of wheat waves and sweeps in the wind. Remember about this, too, for it has something to do with the very beginning of the baby.

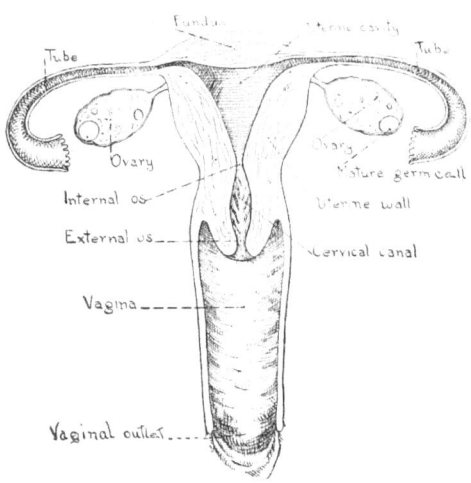

Fig. 3.—Diagram showing the structure and relation of the female generative organs, as seen from the front.

The Ovaries. Very near and a little below the flaring, open ends of the tubes are the ovaries, the sex glands of the female. There is one on each side, held in place by ligaments and they are about the size and shape of almonds. In the ovaries are embedded the *ova*, or eggs, the female germ cells which are concerned with producing the baby and also with the function of menstruation.

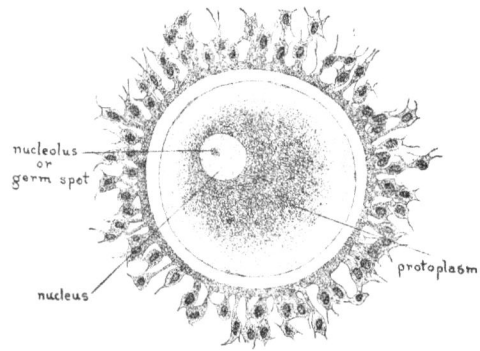

Fig. 4.—Diagram of human ovum.

Just a word about what is meant by "a cell." It is simply a tiny mass of jelly-like substance, called protoplasm, contained in a thin membrane or skin and is so small that it can be seen only through a microscope. In its unmatured state the ovum is a single cell, about $\frac{1}{125}$ of an inch in diameter. In the protoplasm there is a spot called the nucleus and within this a smaller one called the nucleolus, or the germinal spot. These are long names and you need not remember them unless you want to, but glance at Fig. 4 which shows an ovum and you will see that in its general structure it is much like a hen's egg, for the latter has a yolk within the white and on the yolk a tiny speck or germinal spot. The formation of each woman's full quota of ova, fifty thousand or more, is probably complete at the time of her birth.

The vagina is a muscular tube, or passage way, leading from the outside of the body to the cervix, which you will remember is the lower part of the uterus. The vagina slopes upward from its opening and instead of meeting the cervix evenly it meets it almost at right angles and encases it like a sheath for about half an inch. Fig. 2 shows how these organs would appear if we were looking at them from the side.

The Bladder. If you will glance again at Fig. 2, you will see that just in front of the vagina there is a tiny passage leading up to a sac which also is in front of the vagina, and since in this picture it is practically empty, it lies below the uterus. This sac is the bladder and you can readily understand that as the uterus enlarges during pregnancy, it presses upon the bladder and this pressure on the outside gives the same sensation as is produced by pressure from the inside when the bladder is filled with urine. That is why the expectant mother has such a constant desire to urinate during the early weeks of pregnancy, before the uterus pushes up into the abdomen, and also during the later weeks, as well as during labor, when the bladder is being pressed upon by the baby's head.

The Rectum. In the same picture you will see the rectum which lies just behind the uterus and vagina and which terminates in the *anus*. Between the rectum and the vagina is a thick triangular mass of muscle, called the *perineum*, which practically forms a floor to the pelvis, the bony basin without a bottom.

The external genitalia, sometimes called the *vulva*, really have nothing to do with the creation of the baby, but you will better understand some of the care that is given you if you know a little about them, too. Between the thighs, where they join the body, are two thick folds of flesh, called the *labia* and between these lie the perineum, just mentioned, and the openings from the rectum, vagina and bladder as shown in Fig. 2.

Now that we have something of an idea of the structure of the organs concerned with the creation of the baby, we shall want to learn about the usual activities of these interesting little parts, before the baby begins his life within them.

Puberty or Adolescence. You know, of course, that girls are incapable of becoming mothers until after what is termed puberty, or adolescence, and by these terms we mean the period during which childhood develops into sexual maturity, and the individual becomes capable of reproduction. The age at which puberty occurs varies with climate, race and occupation and with different individuals of the same status. But the average for girls, in temperate climates, is from the twelfth to the sixteenth year and for boys from the fourteenth to the seventeenth year. Girls in southern climates sometimes mature as early as the eighth or ninth year while in colder regions puberty may be delayed until they are eighteen or twenty years old.

The occurrence of puberty marks the establishment of *ovulation* and *menstruation*, two functions which are usually performed once a month during the childbearing period.

Ovulation, which probably occurs about midway between the menstrual periods, is simply the name which has been given to the principal function of the ovary and may be defined as the development of the ovum, or egg, and its expulsion, when mature, from the ovary. As the entire human body has its origin in this tiny ovum, its career and course of development are of momentous importance to us, and at the same time furnish a tale of absorbing interest. The ovaries are packed full of these tiny egg-like cells, which probably lie dormant, as stated before, until the girl reaches puberty. Then they begin to develop and grow and push their way from the inside of the ovary to the surface where they look more or less like blisters. When an ovum reaches the surface of the ovary, a thin membrane which contains it, bursts, and it is suddenly expelled into the abdominal cavity. You will remember that the ovary is very near the funnel-like end of the tube, so, when the little cell is shot out of the ovary, it finds itself floating around quite close to this wide opening. Some of the ova that are projected into the abdominal cavity are doubtless lost, but others find their way into the near-by mouth of the tube, and if not fertilized by uniting with a male cell, which we shall explain presently, they pass down the tube into the uterus and are finally carried out in the menstrual flow. It is probable that as a rule only one ovum ripens and escapes from the ovary each month from puberty until the menopause or change of life.

The interesting thing about all of this is that each time an ovum does mature and is discharged from the ovary, the lining of the uterus becomes thicker and softer in order to facilitate the attachment of the ovum, if it is fertilized, this attachment being necessary if a baby is to develop. This preparation of the uterine lining is often, and very appropriately, referred to as "nest-building."

Menstruation, which is the evidence of sexual maturity, is a monthly hemorrhage from the uterus, escaping through the vagina, and it normally recurs regularly throughout the childbearing period, except during pregnancy and while the young mother nurses her baby. The length of this childbearing period is about thirty years and continues from puberty until the menopause. The frequency of the menstrual periods varies from twenty-one to thirty days but the normal interval between periods is twenty-eight days, which is the length of what is called the "menstrual cycle." Thus it is usually a lunar month from the beginning of one period to the next one, making thirteen menstrual periods during each calendar year. The complete course of a menstrual cycle consists of four stages, which, it is believed, occur somewhat as follows:

The first, or constructive stage, lasts about seven days. It is during this stage that the preparations are made to receive the ovum traveling down the tube. The entire uterus becomes congested with blood and is somewhat enlarged and softened as a result, while its lining grows red, thick and velvety. If the ovum remains unfertilized, which is usually the case, it does not attach itself to this elaborately prepared lining, but passes out with the uterine discharges and all of this preparation not only goes for naught but must be undone.

The second stage, therefore, which lasts about five days, is the **destructive stage** and is the period we speak of as menstruation. During this period the extra tissue which has been formed in the uterus is broken down; it mixes with the blood that oozes from the congested lining and together they pour from the vagina as the menstrual flow.

The third or reparative stage, which follows, occupies about three days during which time the uterus and its lining return to their normal state.

The fourth, or quiescent stage, now follows and lasts twelve or fourteen days. This is the time remaining before Nature, with unwearying patience, begins all over again to prepare for the reception and attachment of the next matured ovum, in ease of its possible fertilization. And so it goes, month after month and year after year.

It is very important for a woman who is suffering from painful menstruation to consult a doctor about correcting the cause, in the interests of her future childbearing, if for no other reason, for this is one step toward preparing a good soil in which to plant the seed from which a baby may grow. For example, a misplacement of the uterus is a frequent cause of painful menstruation and if it remains uncorrected may make conception impossible; or if conception perchance does take place, the malposition of the uterus may, later, be the cause of an abortion or miscarriage. Inflammation of the lining of the uterus is another cause of menstrual difficulty and if allowed to persist, may interfere later on with the normal development and nourishment of the baby.

The **menopause**, also termed the climacteric, or the change of life, marks the permanent stopping of menstruation and ability to bear children. This ordinarily occurs between the ages of forty and fifty, the majority of women ceasing to menstruate during their forty-sixth year.

The most favorable age for motherhood to begin is a subject of considerable interest to most women. When it is considered from all standpoints, social, ethical, spiritual as well as physical, the most favorable age for motherhood to begin seems to be sometime in the early twenties. Children have been born to little girls nine years old and to women over sixty, but the extremes of the reproductive years are not favorable periods for childbearing.

Now a word about the **breasts**. They appear to be merely large, soft masses of fat, one on each side of the chest, having no connection with the pelvic organs. But in reality they are very complicated glands and strangely enough, though no one knows why, their activities are controlled by the activities of the generative organs down in the pelvis. Certain it is that their function is very important to the baby, for the breasts are the factories in which nourishment is produced to nourish him during the first few months after he is born.

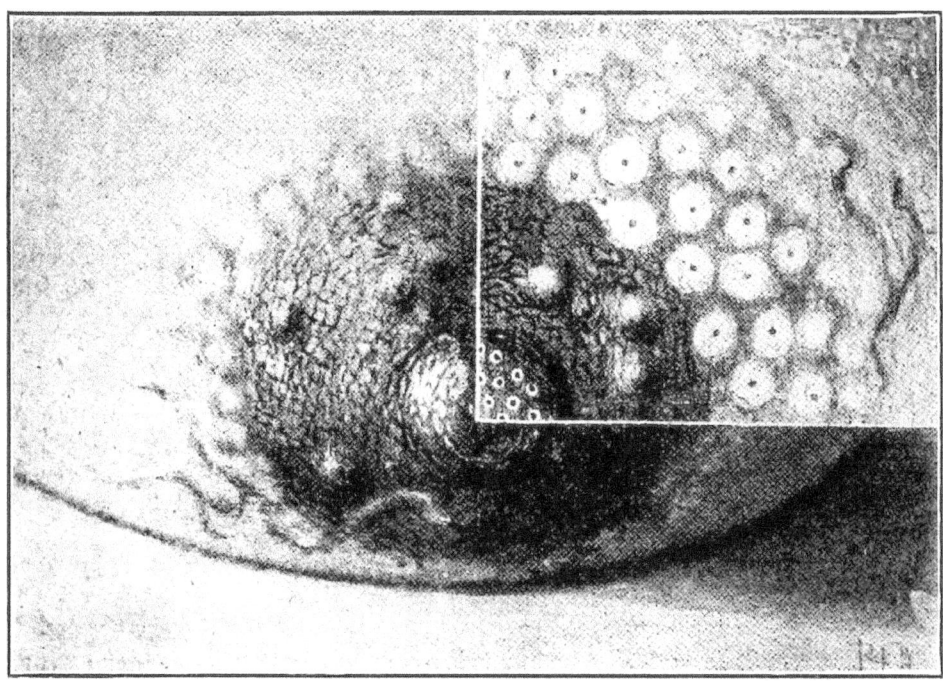

Fig. 5.—Front view of breast, showing areola; openings from milk ducts and the glands beneath the skin.

If we could look inside of the breasts we should see that in structure they are much like several clusters of grapes in which the stems and grapes are hollow. The milk is formed in the tiny sacs corresponding to the grapes, and pours into the little tubes conforming to the stems; these empty into a central tube, opening upon the surface of the nipple from which the baby will extract his nourishment. If you will look at Fig. 5 you will see in that picture of the front of a breast, that a part of it apparently has been magnified to show these openings of the milk ducts. There are about fifteen or twenty of them in each nipple. The picture shows also the little glands which appear as small lumps under the skin around the nipple, both in the dark circle called the *areola* and in the white skin surrounding it.

Summing up this chapter briefly, we find that the pelvis is an irregular, bony canal or basin, drawn in about the middle, thus forming the upper, or false pelvis and lower or true pelvis, neither of which has a bottom. The opening between these two basins is called the inlet, while the lower margin of the true pelvis is called the outlet, but it is the inlet that is of particular importance during childbirth. In the center of the lower pelvis and swung upon ligaments attached to its sides is the uterus, whose lower part, called the cervix, extends downward into the vagina; while reaching out from the upper corners of the uterus are the tubes, and near their open ends, one on each side, are the ovaries filled with germ cells called ova. The bladder lies in front of the uterus and vagina and the rectum behind, while below is the perineum, forming a floor to the pelvic cavity. Every four weeks during the childbearing years an ovum is expelled from one of the ovaries into the abdominal cavity and the uterus regularly prepares to receive it in case of its fertilization, but if it is not fertilized the ovum is lost and menstruation occurs.

We see, too, that although the breasts are situated remotely from the pelvic organs they are really very important accessories, since they provide milk to nourish the baby after his life within the uterus is terminated by his birth.

CHAPTER IV
HOW THE BABY DEVELOPS BEFORE HE IS BORN

Now that we know something of the place where the baby's life begins and how the way is prepared for his growth, we are ready to follow the interesting course of events that occur from the time the seed, a tiny egg-like cell, bursts from an ovary until the beautiful, fully developed baby comes into the world.

You will remember that when the ovum is expelled from an ovary it may float about in the abdominal cavity and be lost or it may enter the near-by mouth of a tube. Also that if it enters a tube it is carried downward toward the uterine cavity by the sweeping motion of the hair-like projections on the lining of the tube. This journey of the ovum through the tube is of enormous consequence, for during its course occur the events which decide whether the ovum shall, like most of its fellows, be simply swept along to no end and lost, or whether by chance it is to receive the mysterious impulse which begins the development of a new human being. The amazing power which enables this cell to reproduce itself, and to develop with unbelievable complexity is acquired somewhere in the tube, usually in the upper end, by meeting and fusing with a *spermatozoon*, the germinal cell of the male.

The spermatozoa are attracted to the ovum much as bits of metal are drawn to a magnet, but although the ovum that is destined to be fertilized is surrounded by several spermatozoa, only one actually enters and fuses with it.

This fusion is termed **fertilization**, or, in lay parlance, **conception**, and the instant at which it occurs marks the beginning of pregnancy. The establishment of this fact is of considerable importance, since it does away with any possible controversy concerning the time at which a new life begins. The origin of the baby is exactly coincident with the fusion of the male and female cells. Furthermore, the sex of the child and any inherited traits and characteristics are also established at this decisive moment. No amount of dieting, exercise or mental effort on the part of the expectant mother can alter or influence them in the smallest degree, for the father has made his complete contribution toward the creation of the new being and the mother, also, has made hers, except for nourishment which she provides throughout pregnancy.

All told, probably more than five hundred theories have been advanced to explain what it is that decides of which sex the forthcoming child is going to be. But as the results of applying these theories have scarcely borne out the claims of their advocates, they are given but scant attention to-day.

The present belief regarding the causation of sex is that although there is but one kind of ovum, there are two kinds of spermatozoa, one capable of producing a male and the other a female child, but the sex-determining form of the male cell that fertilizes any one ovum is a matter of the merest chance. Statistics show that more male than female babies are born, the usual proportion being about 105 boys to 100 girls among those who are carried to "term" or the end of pregnancy. Among abortions and prematurely born babies there is also a larger number of boys than girls, but as more boys than girls die in infancy, the two sexes about even up in the number of those living to adult life.

Concerning the time of the month when conception is most likely to occur, there is a wide difference of opinion. Some doctors think that the most favorable period is just before or just after menstruation, while others believe that conception is most likely to take place about midway between the menstrual periods.

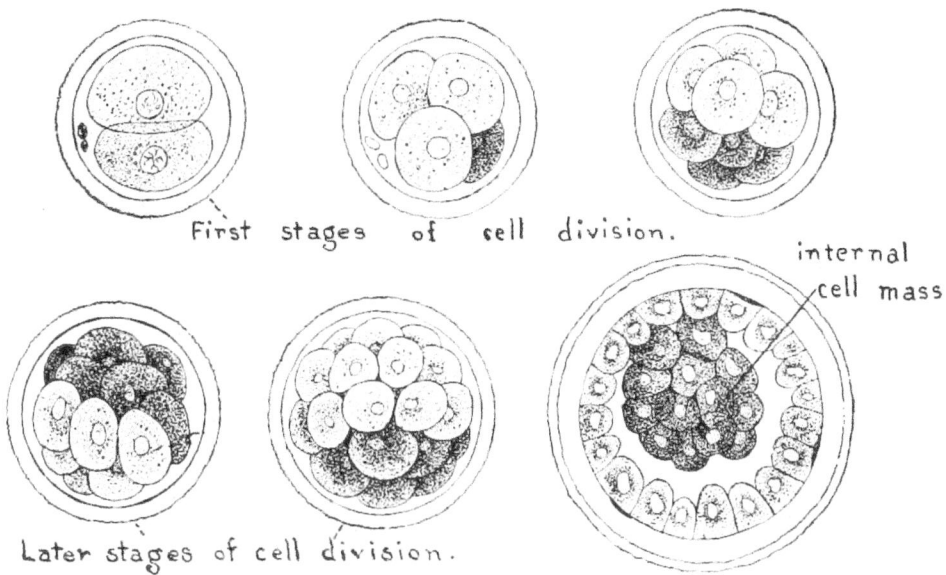

Fig. 6.—Diagram indicating process of cell division.

Returning to the ovum which meets a spermatozoon in the course of its journey down the tube, we find that as soon as a spermatozoon enters an ovum it disappears and is completely absorbed, and, as the ovum in turn is instantly possessed of new powers, through the presence of the male cell, the result of this union is an entirely new cell. But instead of continuing its existence as a single cell, the fertilized ovum divides into two cells; these two into four; the four into eight and so on until a clustering mass of cells is formed which looks something like a mulberry. If you will look at Fig. 6 you will see what happens as this cell division progresses and also that in time the cells rearrange themselves in such a way as to leave a space in the center of the mass so that it becomes a little sac with a cluster of cells at one point, which hangs toward the center, called the *internal cell mass*. This will interest you because it is from cells at one point in this little cluster that the baby begins to develop, together with the cord, bag of waters and afterbirth, to be described later.

While these changes are taking place, the entire mass is being carried slowly down the tube toward the uterus by the sweeping motion of the soft little hairs on the lining of the tube. It is steadily growing, and by the time it reaches the uterus the mass is about the size of the head of a pin. As you will remember, the lining of the uterus prepares each month to receive the fertilized ovum, becoming soft and thick. The cell mass floats around for a little while after it reaches the uterine cavity and then resting at some point, sinks down into the soft lining and is completely buried.

From now on the cells which compose the mass rapidly increase in number and very shortly cease to be all of one kind. These different kinds of cells rearrange themselves and grow in such a manner that some of them begin to form the different parts of the baby's body and others develop into two thin membranes that finally enclose the baby in a double sac. He is attached to the inner surface of the sac; the space which he does not occupy is filled with fluid and the sac itself is attached to the uterine lining at the point where the cell mass happened to stop and bury itself.

This sac is what you have heard called the "bag of waters," but the doctors refer to it as the **membranes**. As it enlarges and pushes out into the uterine cavity it still consists of two thin membranes except where it is attached to the uterus, at which point it grows into a thick, spongy mass of blood-vessels. These blood-vessels divide and branch out in a tree-like fashion and burrow into the uterine wall. As you will see later, it is through this mass of branching blood-vessels that the baby virtually eats and breathes and gives off waste materials during the nine months of his life within the uterus. The doctors refer to the mass as the **placenta** but you have heard it called the "afterbirth," because it is expelled after the baby is born.

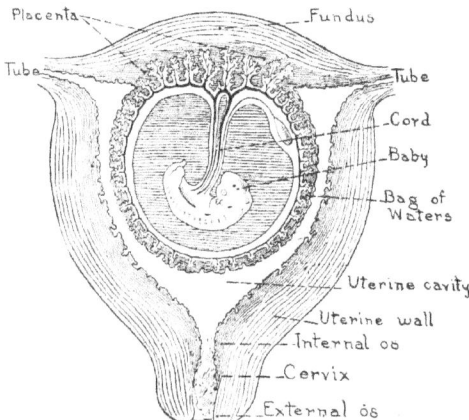

Fig. 7.—Diagram showing the developing baby, at an early stage, with cord, membranes and placenta, within the uterine cavity.

As the baby's development advances the part by which he is connected with the placenta lengthens out into what is called the **umbilical cord**. There are blood-vessels in this cord through which blood constantly flows back and forth, carrying nourishment to the baby from his mother and waste matter from his little body to the placenta where it is taken up by her blood. But this exchange of materials takes place through thin membranes and consequently the blood of the mother and baby never mingle. Fig. 7 will give you an idea of how the sac of membranes, with the baby hanging inside, grows out into the uterine cavity; how at the point where the membranes are attached to the uterus the blood-vessels have developed into the thick, spongy placenta and how the baby is connected with it by means of the cord. In Fig. 8 you may see how the baby changes in appearance as the weeks of pregnancy go by. At the end of the fourth month he really looks quite like the baby that we are so eagerly preparing for.

If we follow his development within the uterus month by month, we find that **by the end of the first lunar month, or fourth week**, the baby's body is about ½ inch long and looks about as is suggested in the third little outline in Fig. 8.

At the end of the second month, or eighth week, his head is fairly well shaped; bones are beginning to develop, webbed hands and feet are formed and the little body is about 1 inch long.

At the end of the third month, or twelfth week, his entire body shows marked development and is about 3½ inches long. His fingers and toes are separated and bear soft nails; the teeth are forming, the eyes have lids and the umbilical cord has taken definite form.

At the end of the fourth month, or sixteenth week, in addition to the development of all parts a fine, soft hair appears over the body; there is a black, tarry substance, called *meconium*, in the baby's intestines and he measures about 6 inches in length and weighs perhaps ¼ pound.

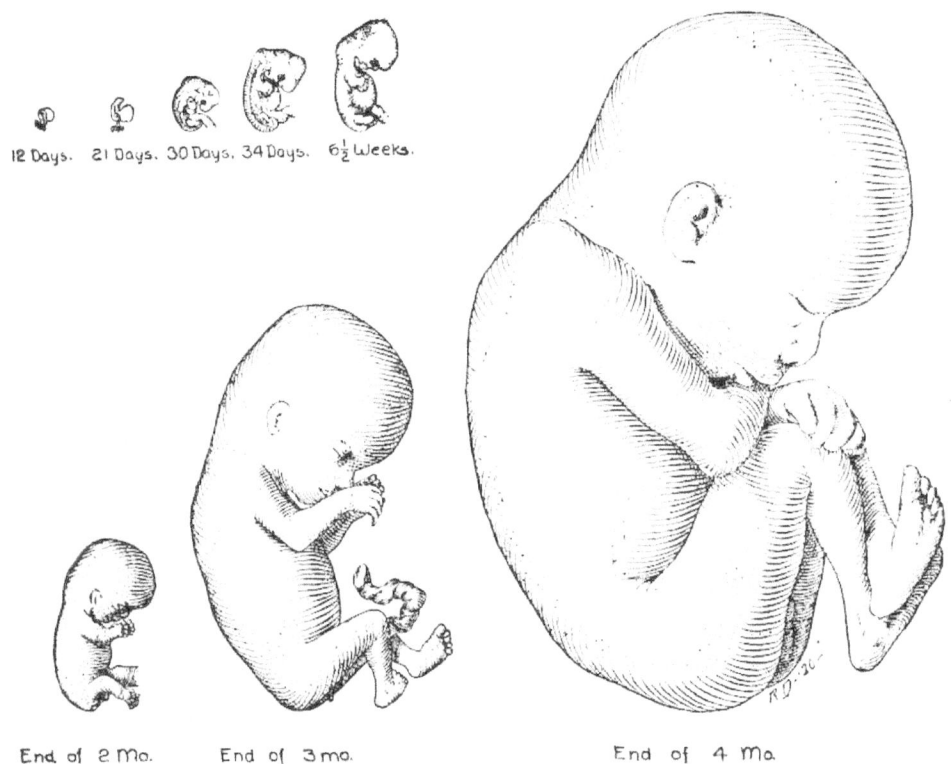

Fig. 8.—Appearance of the baby at different stages, early in his development.

By the end of the fifth month, or twentieth week, the baby has grown and developed markedly. He is now covered with skin on which are occasional patches of a greasy, cheesy substance called *vernix caseosa*, and though there is some fat beneath the skin his face looks old and wrinkled. A certain amount of hair has appeared upon the head and the eyelids are opening. It is usually during the fifth month that the expectant mother first feels her baby move, this sensation being commonly referred to as "quickening." He is now about 10 inches long and weighs about 9 ounces.

By the end of the sixth month or twenty-fourth week, the baby is about 12 inches long and weighs possibly 1½ pounds. He is thin and wrinkled in appearance and if born at this time will attempt to breathe and move his limbs but will perish in a short time.

By the end of the seventh month, or twenty-eighth week, he still looks thin and scrawny; his skin is reddish and is well covered with the cheesy vernix caseosa. If born at this stage, the baby will move quite vigorously and cry feebly, but he is not likely to live for any length of time. He is now about 14 inches long and weighs about 2¾ pounds.

By the end of the eighth month, or thirty-second week, the baby has grown to about 17 inches in length and 4 pounds in weight, but continues to look thin and old and wrinkled. His nails do not extend beyond the ends of his fingers but are firmer in texture; the soft, downy hair begins to disappear from his face but the hair on his head is more abundant. If born at this stage, the baby will have a fair chance to live, provided he is given painstaking care. This is true in spite of the old belief, still widely current, that a seven months' baby is more likely to live than one born at eight months (meaning calendar months). The fact is that after the twenty-eighth week the probability of the baby's living increases greatly with each added week of life within the uterus. His growth during the latter part of pregnancy is rapid, for he gains nine tenths of his weight after the fifth month and one half of his weight during the last eight weeks of uterine life.

At the end of the ninth month, or thirty-sixth week, the increased amount of fat under the baby's skin has given a plumper, rounder contour to the entire body; the aged look has passed and his chances for life have greatly increased. He weighs about 5½ pounds at this stage and is perhaps 18 inches long.

The end of the tenth month, or fortieth week, usually marks the end of pregnancy. Fig. 9 will show you how the baby lies in the uterus just before birth, curled up into the smallest possible space.

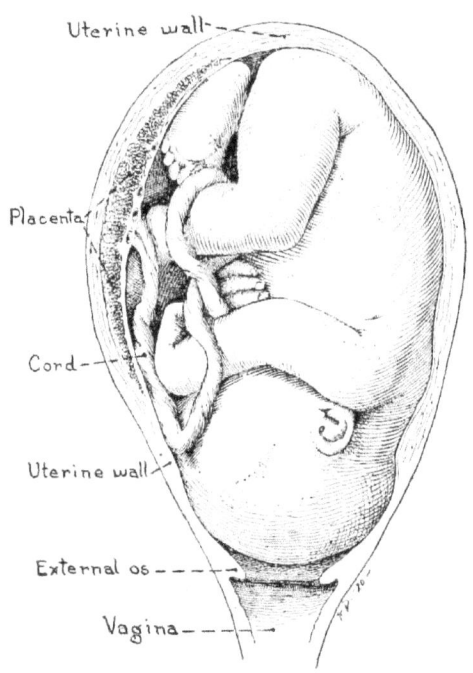

FIG. 9.—The usual position of the baby just before he is born.

The average normally developed baby has grown to a length of about 20 inches and weighs about 7¼ pounds, boys usually being about three ounces heavier than girls, but there may be a variation of weight among entirely normal, healthy babies from a minimum of 5 pounds to as high as 11 pounds or more. Newborn babies very seldom weigh more than 12 pounds, in spite of legends and rumors to the contrary.

The size of the baby is affected by the race of his parents; colored babies, for example, averaging a smaller weight than white babies. And, as might be expected, the size of the parents is likely to be reflected in their infants, large parents tending to have large children and vice versa.

The number of children which the mother has previously borne is also a factor, since the first child is usually the smallest, the size of those following showing an increase with the mother's age up to her twenty-eighth year, if her pregnancies do not occur at too frequent intervals.

Twins. Sometimes a woman gives birth to more than one baby at the same time. When there are two they are called twins; triplets when there are three; quadruplets, quintuplets and sextuplets respectively, when there are four, five and six babies within the uterus at once. Six is the largest accredited number on record.

It is estimated that twins occur once in ninety pregnancies and triplets once in about seven thousand cases. The tendency seems to be inherited, as is evidenced by the number of twins and triplets to be found among relatives.

Twins are often prematurely born and each is likely to be smaller than a baby resulting from a single pregnancy, but their combined weight is greater than the weight of one normal baby.

Extra-uterine Pregnancy. Another departure from the normal pregnancy is when the baby develops outside of the uterus. Although in the normal course of events the fertilized ovum travels down the tube and becomes attached to the uterine lining, it is possible for it to stop, and more or less completely develop at any point along the way. This is called an extra-uterine pregnancy, since it occurs outside of the uterus. If the baby develops in one of the ovaries, it is termed an ovarian pregnancy, and a tubal pregnancy if it develops in a tube, this being the most frequent variety of extra-uterine pregnancies. Only about one out of a hundred such pregnancies continue throughout the allotted period, and accordingly, a live baby, capable of living for any length of time, seldom results.

To sum up a normal pregnancy, we find that in the course of ten lunar months following the fertilization of an ovum, the uterus grows from a small, flattened pelvic organ, 3 inches in length, to a large muscular sac, about 15 inches long occupying the abdominal cavity. It increases its weight sixteen times, that is, from 2 ounces to 2 pounds, while the capacity of the uterine cavity is multiplied five hundred times. Within the uterus is a baby weighing about 7¼ pounds; a placenta weighing perhaps 1¼ pounds and approximately a quart of fluid. The baby is attached to the placenta by means of a jelly-like cord about as thick as one's first finger and 20 inches long; baby, placenta, cord and fluid all being contained in a thin, but strong sac frequently called the bag of waters, but by the doctors termed the membranes. The total weight of the uterus and its contents at the end of pregnancy is usually about 15 pounds.

Throughout the baby's life within the uterus, the placenta virtually acts as his digestive organs, lungs, kidneys and bowels. Bear this in mind, and you will realize why, in taking care of yourself you are taking care of your baby while his body is being built and getting itself into running order to take up life as a separate being. The full realization that whatever is good for you is good for your baby will make you eager to give yourself the care that is outlined in the next chapter.

CHAPTER V
TAKING CARE OF THE BABY BEFORE HE COMES

We shall see that taking care of your baby before he is born means taking such care of yourself throughout pregnancy, that you not only keep your own body in its usual good running order, but in addition, so effectively promote the activities of your various organs that you also keep the baby's body going, his body that is growing all the time.

Quite reasonably this requires extra work on the part of some of your organs, particularly those concerned with digestion and the process of throwing off impurities. The latter is of the greatest possible importance for in addition to excreting the usual amount of impurities from your own body you must excrete also those thrown off by your baby. The amount of waste from him is not large but it seems to be of such a character that it harms the mother if it is not steadily excreted.

Good digestion and satisfactory excretion are dependent upon a number of factors and fortunately most of them are within your own control.

Your frame of mind is one of the most important factors of all. I know that to suggest the cultivation of a cheerful, hopeful mental attitude is easier said than done. But after all it really is largely a matter of habit which you can acquire if you set yourself to it, particularly if you realize that your physical condition will be benefited by your going through pregnancy happily. And remember that whatever is good for you is good for your baby.

Continue with the work, amusements and exercise that you are used to and enjoy, except of course such activities as the doctor may forbid. In general, try to forget that you are pregnant, so far as you can do this and still remember to take proper care of yourself.

Above all, don't worry. Worry will interfere with your sleep and it will also upset your digestion quite as seriously as will wrong food. Try not to be too self-centered or too watchful of your symptoms, but at the same time avoid the dangerous habit of thinking that any unusual condition which develops is due to your being pregnant, for a sick pregnancy is not normal.

It will relieve you of a great deal of anxiety if you report to your doctor everything you do not understand, for the consciousness that he will know just what to do, if anything is necessary, will help to keep you from worrying.

It is important, too, for you to get rid of the depressing beliefs in connection with pregnancy that have come down to us through the ages.

For instance, do not believe for a moment that anything you do, think or see can "mark" or deform your baby, for remember that after conception you give him nothing but nourishment. The only communication between you and the baby is through your and his blood, and blood does not carry mental impressions. Accordingly, no effects of fear, horror or unpleasant memories which you may have can possibly reach him. It is true that once in a while a woman does see something shocking and later gives birth to a marked or deformed baby. But there is little doubt, now, that such an occurrence is merely a coincidence. If you will stop and think for a moment you will realize that most expectant mothers see or hear or think something unpleasant at some time during pregnancy, and yet most babies are born without mark or blemish. Anger, fright or sudden shock may upset your digestion, but it does not directly affect your baby.

As for that common belief that in "reaching up" the mother may slip the cord around the baby's neck—if you will picture for a moment how the baby lies within the uterus you will realize how impossible this is, for the mother's arms have no connection with him or the cord.

So dismiss these doubts and fears from your mind and dwell instead upon the loveliness of what is in store for you, for, I repeat, your physical condition will be benefited if you go through pregnancy happily. And remember again that whatever is good for you is good for your baby.

So your first step toward caring for the little life already within your charge is to follow the example of Mrs. Wiggs, who constantly wiped the dust from her rose-colored spectacles.

Now for the more specific details of your care. Of these the question of your **diet** is of enormous importance.

Let us consider first what your food accomplishes if it is suitable and conditions are favorable for its use by you and the baby. It should provide nourishment for your various tissues, as under ordinary conditions; it should promote the activities of your skin and kidneys, as well as bowels, since it is through them that the waste from your own and your baby's body must be excreted, and your food should be adequate also, to build and nourish the baby's body without his having to draw materials from your tissues. Strange as it may seem, the baby's physical needs are supplied before yours are met, and if there are not enough food materials for you both, your bones, teeth and muscles will be deprived. Furthermore, taking proper food during pregnancy is an important step toward preparing yourself to nurse your baby, after he is born, which is quite as urgent as nourishing him before birth.

To accomplish these ends you not only must eat suitable food, but you must digest and absorb it as well. This requires that you constantly guard against overeating, constipation and indigestion of any kind. Indigestion may be avoided during pregnancy exactly as it is at other times, by eating proper food, by cultivating a happy frame of mind; by having sufficient exercise, fresh air, rest and sleep.

If you are accustomed to a fairly simple, well balanced, mixed diet, you probably will need to make little or no change, except to have the evening meal light if it has been a hearty one. It may surprise you to learn that you need not "eat for two," in quantity, as is so commonly believed necessary, for during pregnancy you make so much better use of food materials than usual that an amount and kind of food that keep you in good condition will be adequate to meet your baby's needs, too, until the latter part of pregnancy. On the other hand, it is very unwise for an expectant mother to cut down her diet, with the idea of keeping the baby small and thus make labor easy, except under the direction of her doctor. In general it is the size of the baby's head that makes labor easy or difficult, and not the amount of fat distributed over his body. And if the mother cuts down the minerals in her diet to make the baby bones soft, the only result is that her own bones and teeth are softened, because the baby extracts from them enough lime to supply what the food lacks.

Three meals a day will usually be enough during at least the first half of pregnancy and they should be taken with clock-like regularity, eaten slowly and masticated thoroughly. The possible need for slight additional food during the later weeks may be supplied more satisfactorily by lunches of milk, cocoa or broth and crackers or toast, between meals and upon retiring, than by taking larger meals. An expectant mother who has a tendency to nausea early in pregnancy often feels better for taking a small lunch regularly five or six times daily instead of the usual three full meals.

It is of the greatest importance that every pregnant woman drink an abundance of fluid to act as a solvent for her food and waste material and promote the activity of her kidneys, skin and bowels. She needs about three quarts daily, most of which should be water, the remainder consisting of milk, cocoa, soup and other liquids. Alcohol should not be taken except upon the doctor's orders and only moderate amounts of coffee and tea, unless he gives permission for more.

The expectant mother will be wise to avoid fried food, pastry, rich desserts, rich salad dressings and any other food which would ordinarily disagree with her.

Since the enjoyment of one's meals promotes digestion at all times, the expectant mother should try to eat the things that she enjoys most and that agree with her. The average pregnant woman who has no symptoms of complications will usually be able to supply her own and her baby's needs and at the same time keep within the bounds of safety if she selects her diet from the foods included in the following groups:

Animal Foods. Milk and eggs are the most satisfactory, but for the sake of variety and to tempt her appetite the expectant mother will usually be allowed to take rather sparingly, and preferably only once a day, of fish, the various kinds of shell fish, beef, lamb, chicken or game. Pork, veal and goose should be avoided as a rule, and particularly by women with whom they ordinarily disagree.

Soups. Thin soups and broths have little food value but because of their appetizing flavor and aroma are an aid to digestion, and frequently by stimulating a flagging appetite will help the expectant mother to eat and assimilate more than she would without them. But cream soups and purées have a high food value and, like thin soups and broths, also supply a definite amount of fluid which she must have.

Vegetables. The group of vegetables generally designated as "leafy" are of even greater importance to the expectant mother than they are to the average person. Of these she may safely eat onions, asparagus, celery, string beans, spinach, and she should make a point of taking a green salad, such as lettuce, cress or romaine, at least once daily. Sweet potatoes, white potatoes, rice, peas, Lima beans, tomatoes, beets and carrots, also, may be eaten with safety, as a rule, but cabbage, cauliflower, corn, egg-plant, Brussels sprouts, parsnips, cucumbers and radishes should be taken with great caution and avoided altogether if they cause gas or any kind of distress.

Fresh Fruits. A necessary part of the diet is fresh fruit, and among those fruits which are both beneficial and usually harmless are apples, peaches, apricots, pears, oranges, figs, cherries, pineapple, grapes, plums, strawberries, raspberries, blackberries and grapefruit. These are more likely to be laxative if eaten alone, as before breakfast and at bedtime. Cooked fruits are also valuable articles of diet, but are probably less laxative than raw fruit. Some of the citrous fruits, oranges, grapefruit or lemons, should be taken daily because they possess a certain indispensable food value which is peculiar to them.

Cereals. For their nourishing and laxative qualities, cereals are important and their food value is increased by the milk and cream which are usually taken with them. Cooked cereals should invariably be cooked longer than the usual directions suggest. Bran, eaten alone as a cereal or in combination with other grains, is an excellent laxative.

Breads. Graham, cornmeal, whole wheat and bran bread are all good, in general the expectant mother will be on the safe side if she eats sparingly, if at all, of very fresh or hot breads and hot cakes.

Desserts. Desserts are very important for they add to the attractiveness of most people's meals, and if wisely chosen and properly made, may supply a good deal of easily digested nourishment. They may include, in addition to fresh and cooked fruits and preserves, ice-cream, a wide variety of custards, creams and puddings made largely of milk, eggs and some ingredient to give substance and firmness, such as gelatin, cornstarch, rice, tapioca, farina, arrow-root and similar materials.

In general the expectant mother should eat an abundance of fruit and vegetables, taking at least some uncooked fruit and a green salad, daily, and make sure that her food contains a good deal of residue, such as is provided by fruit and coarse vegetables. This residue increases the bulk of the material in the intestines, and this helps to overcome the tendency toward constipation. As fat is less easily digested than starchy foods, and more likely to cause nausea during pregnancy, it is better to eat no more fat than usual but to supply the additional material which is needed after about the sixth month, by taking a little more starchy food. However, a slight increase only is necessary, and this chiefly during the last three or four weeks.

The Kidneys. It is scarcely possible to say enough about the importance of keeping your kidneys in normal working order during pregnancy, for through them is excreted much of the waste matter from your baby's body as well as your own. Sometimes when these impurities are not thrown off as they should be the expectant mother has convulsions. You will be glad to know how much you yourself can do toward preventing convulsions by drinking plenty of water and by faithfully measuring your urine and taking a specimen to the doctor when he asks you to. As I said before, you should drink at least three quarts of fluid every day. Most of this should be water, the remainder being milk, cocoa, soup, tea, coffee, and so on.

The doctor will probably want you to measure your urine and take a specimen to him once a month during the first half of pregnancy and every two weeks afterward, or even every week toward the end. He can tell by examining the urine whether your kidneys are acting as they should and if they are not he may save you serious trouble by putting you to bed for a few days with no nourishment but milk and water.

In preparing a specimen you will need a covered corked vessel large enough to hold all the urine passed in twenty-four hours, and it must be thoroughly washed and scalded. The next step is to pass urine, suppose we say at eight o'clock in the morning, and throw it away. All of the urine which you pass after this time until eight o'clock the next morning must be saved in the vessel and kept in a cool place to prevent its decomposing. If you will put a teaspoonful of chloroform or boracic acid powder into the vessel it will tend to preserve the urine and will not injure the specimen. At the end of twenty-four hours the urine should be shaken to mix it thoroughly and about half a pint poured into a bottle that has been washed and scalded. Carefully cork and label this with the date, your name and address and the total amount of urine passed in the twenty-four hours. The vessel for collecting the urine and whatever you use as a measure should be reserved for these purposes only. If you have no tin or glass measure, a regular-size quart tomato can will prove entirely satisfactory.

If you find, when measuring your urine, that you pass less than a quart and a half in twenty-four hours, you may know without being told that this is not enough and that you should drink more water.

The Skin. People are likely to think of the skin as being simply a covering for the body, whereas, in reality, it is a very complicated and active organ which helps to regulate the body temperature and constantly throws off impurities, just as the kidneys do. This latter function is performed by the sweat glands which open upon the surface of the skin as the "pores," and we are told that in all there are some twenty-eight miles of these tiny tube-like structures in the skin. These glands should be, and usually are, constantly active; they pour upon the surface of the body an oily substance which keeps the skin soft; they also excrete something more than a pint of water daily, which contains impurities that are harmful if retained in the body. We are not aware of this constant excretion of fluids, which is termed "insensible perspiration," but it continues even in cold weather and must not be stopped if health is to be preserved. If the oil, dust, particles of dead skin and the waste material left by dried perspiration are allowed to remain upon the surface of the body they will clog the pores, or gland openings, and thus interfere with their action. The removal of this material, then, is necessary to maintain health, and is done automatically in part for the fluid evaporates and much of the solid matter is rubbed off on the clothing. The most important aids to the skin's activity are the drinking of plenty of water, deep breathing, exercise and warm baths.

Regular and thorough bathing serves the double purpose of removing waste matter already on the surface, and of stimulating the glands to increased activity in giving off still more.

Many doctors advise a warm, not hot, shower or tub bath every day, with soap used freely over the entire body, followed by a brisk rub. The best time for this warm, cleansing bath, as a rule, is just before retiring, as it is soothing and restful, and tends to induce sleep. Very hot baths are fatiguing, particularly during pregnancy, and should never be taken except with the doctor's permission; but cold baths usually may be continued throughout pregnancy if one is accustomed to them and reacts well afterwards. Under these conditions the morning cold plunge, shower or sponge is beneficial, as it stimulates the circulation and thus promotes the activity of the skin. Some doctors forbid tub bathing of any kind after the seventh month, on the ground that as the expectant mother sits in the tub her vagina is filled with unsterile water and should labor occur shortly afterward an infection, or fever, might result. And as she is heavy and somewhat uncertain on her feet, there is also the danger of her slipping and falling while getting in or out of the tub. Other doctors permit tub baths throughout pregnancy, up until the onset of labor; while as to hot foot baths, since there seems to be no reason for or against them at any time during the nine months, they may be taken or not at will.

Bathing in a quiet stream or lake is apparently harmless but sea bathing, if the surf is rough, is inadvisable because of the beating of the waves upon the abdomen and the general violence of the exercise.

The importance of keeping the body evenly warm throughout pregnancy cannot be overemphasized, for a sudden chilling or wetting may so check action of the skin as to impose more of a burden upon the kidneys than they can meet, in their effort to throw off the skin's share of the body waste. Accordingly, a single chilling will sometimes be enough to cause convulsions. This may be one reason why convulsions occur more frequently during cold weather or after a sudden drop in the temperature after warm or mild days.

The Bowels. The bowels, also, throw off a certain amount of impurities and if they do not move thoroughly at least once a day these impurities may be taken into the system and again the kidneys be given extra work.

Unhappily a great many pregnant women are constipated, particularly during the later weeks, while women who have always had a tendency of this kind may have trouble with their bowels from the very beginning of pregnancy. Your bowels should move regularly every day, and to this end you should attempt to empty them at the same hour each day, immediately after breakfast being the best time. The importance of regularity in making the attempt cannot be overemphasized, even though the bowels do not always move.

The measures which tend to prevent constipation, as already pointed out, are drinking plenty of fluids, and eating fresh fruit, coarse vegetables and bulky cereals such as bran; also taking a glass of hot or cold water just before going to bed and the first thing in the morning. You should not take enemas or cathartics without your doctor's order, but you may safely increase the amount of fluids which you drink and the bulk of your food, in order to regulate your bowels.

Senna and prunes cooked together prove to be helpful in keeping the bowels regular and they are entirely harmless. A simple way of preparing them for this purpose is to pour a quart of boiling water over an ounce of senna leaves and allow them to stand for about two hours. A pound of well washed prunes should soak overnight in this liquor, after it has been strained, and then cooked in it until tender. They may be sweetened with two tablespoonfuls of brown sugar, and the flavor improved by adding a stick of cinnamon or slice of lemon while they are cooking. Half a dozen of these prunes, with some of the syrup, may be taken at the evening meal to start with, and increased or decreased in number as necessary.

Clothes. The chief purpose of clothes under all conditions is to aid in keeping the body warm, thus helping to preserve an even circulation of the blood and the activity of the sweat glands. As has been pointed out, this is of especial importance during pregnancy. The expectant mother's clothes should be not only sufficiently warm, but they should be equally warm over her entire body. They should be light and porous, and fairly loose, so as not to interfere with the circulation or other bodily functions. There must be no pressure on chest or abdomen; no tight garters, belts, collars or shoes.

The clothes of the mother-to-be, like every other detail of her care, must be adapted to her surroundings and mode of living. If her house is well and evenly heated during the cold months, she may quite safely dress lightly while indoors; if it is not, she should wear underwear with high neck, long sleeves and drawers, both indoors and out, except when the weather is warm enough to cause perspiration. At all times, however, the warmth of her clothing should be suited to the temperature of the home, the climate and the state of the weather.

Remembering that it is important for you to keep up the diversions and amusements that you enjoy, it is worth while to have your clothes as pretty and becoming as possible, for you are much more likely to go about and mingle with your friends if you feel that you are becomingly and well dressed. At the same time your clothes should be so made that their weight will hang from the shoulders instead of from the waistband.

And that brings us to the question of **corsets**, a much discussed garment. Women who have not been accustomed to wearing corsets will scarcely feel the need of adopting them during pregnancy except, perhaps, during the later weeks when the heavy abdomen needs to be supported for the sake of comfort. This need is felt particularly by women who have had children and whose abdominal walls are somewhat weakened in consequence.

If you have been wearing comfortable, well fitting corsets, you probably will not feel the need of making a change until the third or fourth month. But by this time the baby will have pushed up out of the lower pelvis into the abdomen and your corsets then, if you wear any, must be so constructed that they will not compress nor disguise your figure, but will provide support and accommodate themselves to an abdomen that is steadily increasing in size and changing in shape. Such corsets are made of soft material; have elastic inserts and have lacings at the sides as well as in the back. They come well down and fit snugly over the hips. (See Fig. 10.) Some women find comfort in attaching shoulder straps to their corsets thus suspending some of the abdominal weight from the shoulders. But as a rule, the most comfortable arrangement is a short-waisted maternity corset worn with a brassière that supports the breasts and does not compress the nipples.

I hope this description will make clear to you why the same style corsets as you ordinarily wear cannot be satisfactory during pregnancy, no matter how large they are, and may even prove harmful.

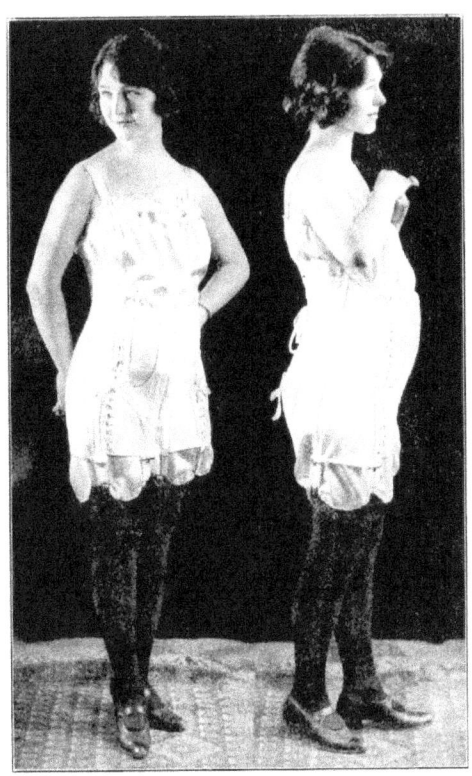

FIG. 10.—Front and side views of a satisfactory maternity corset, adjusted at the fifth month of pregnancy. (By courtesy of Emma E. Goodwin, New York.)

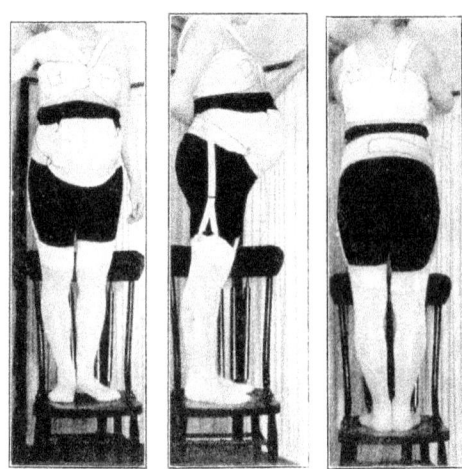

Fig. 11.—Front, side and back views of home-made binder for supporting a heavy, pendulous abdomen during later weeks of pregnancy. It is adjusted as the expectant mother lies down, the ends being crossed in the back and pinned to the lower margin of the front, thus giving additional support.

Also breast-binder made of a straight strip of soft cotton material, 10 or 12 inches wide and 2 yards long. This is crossed in front and held with safety-pins, the ends being carried over the shoulders and pinned to the back of the binder. It should be snug below the breasts but loose over the nipples. The openings over the nipples show how this binder may be used to support the breasts of the nursing mother. (From photographs taken at the Maternity Centre Association, New York.)

Even a properly fitting maternity corset may become uncomfortable during the last few weeks of pregnancy, and have to be replaced by an abdominal supporter of linen or rubber. And when this stage is reached, even the woman who has worn no corsets may find that she is more comfortable if she adopts such a support, particularly at night. There are many admirable binders on the market, or such an one as is illustrated in Figs. 11 and 12 may easily be made at home as well as comfortable and inexpensive stocking supporters, made from tapes or strips of muslin, as in Fig. 13.

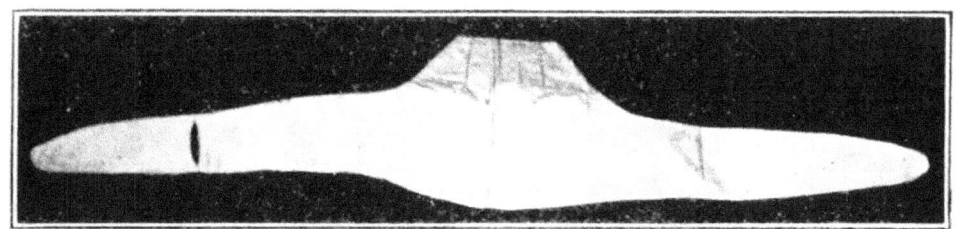

Fig. 12.—Abdominal binder used in Fig. 11, showing darts at top of front to fit it over the abdomen.

Your **shoes**, also, merit some thought, for your feet will probably be larger during the latter part of pregnancy, partly because of the possibility of their being somewhat swollen and partly because the increased weight of your body tends to spread them. This added weight also increases the strain put upon the arch and as a result, flat-foot is fairly common among expectant mothers who have not taken pains to have their arches well supported. Your shoes would better be an inch longer than those you ordinarily wear; they should have broad, common sense heels and fit snugly over the instep, in spite of being full large. If your shoes are not comfortable you will find yourself tiring easily and for this reason will tend to take less exercise than you should.

Another reason for the need of proper shoes is that as pregnancy advances the expectant mother becomes rather unsteady on her feet, and broad, firm heels help to make her feel more secure. The heels need not be flat at first, if you have been accustomed to wearing high ones, for the sudden lowering of the heels may injure your arches, but as the weeks wear on you would better adopt moderately low heels. High French heels should be avoided because they not only increase the difficulty and discomfort of walking but cause backache, as well, by forcing a position that adds to the pressure on the lower part of the abdomen. They increase the risk of turning the ankles, too, and of tripping and falling, which is a very serious accident for the expectant mother.

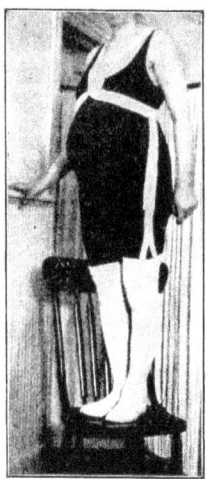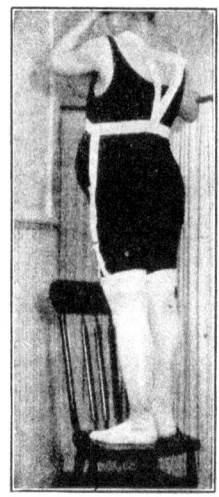

FIG. 13.—Front and back view of home-made stocking supporters made of webbing or 1–inch strips of muslin and a pair of child's side garters. The straps are sewed together in the back, but pinned in front to permit adjustment as the abdomen enlarges. (By courtesy of the Maternity Centre Association, New York.)

Fresh Air. If you realize by this time how important it is to keep your digestion in good order and promote the activity of all your excretory organs, you probably suspect how important fresh air and exercise are to you and your expected baby, because of their effect upon your entire well-being.

The average individual uses up in a minute's time the oxygen contained in four bushels of air, and since the pregnant woman takes in through her lungs the oxygen for both herself and her baby, she must have a sufficient quantity of air to supply at least this amount.

Accordingly, you should make a point of spending at least two hours of each day in the open air. If the weather is so stormy or severe as to make it undesirable for you to go out from under cover, because of the danger of getting wet or chilled, you can wrap up well and take your airing on a protected porch or in a room with all the windows wide open.

But this is only a part of it, for the air in your house or rooms must be kept fresh all day by being constantly changed; this requires a steady inpouring of fresh air and outpouring of stale air.

A very good way to accomplish this is to have one or more windows open slightly, top and bottom, all the time. But there must be no sudden changes of temperature, nor drafts, for fear of chilling your skin. At night you should sleep in a room with the windows open, taking care to be well protected by light, warm coverings.

Exercise. Each detail of the expectant mother's daily routine seems to be more important than the last. And so when we come to the question of regular out-of-door exercise we are almost persuaded to believe that whatever else may be neglected, this is indispensable, since it promotes digestion, stimulates the activity of the skin and lungs, steadies the nerves, quiets the mind and promotes sleep. And more than that, walking, which is probably the most satisfactory form of exercise for her to take, also strengthens some of the muscles that are used during labor. But exercise is downright injurious if continued to the point of fatigue, no matter how little has been taken. Each woman must be a law unto herself in this matter, therefore, and must be impressed with the importance of stopping before she is tired. It may be a good plan for you to start by walking only a short distance at a time, increasing this gradually until you are able to walk possibly as much as an hour in the morning and an hour in the afternoon without fatigue.

All violent exercise and sports are of course to be avoided, particularly swimming, horseback riding and tennis. While motoring and carriage driving are pleasant diversions, they cannot be classed as exercise. They should be taken only in comfortable vehicles and over smooth roads, so that there will be no jarring nor jolting, and the expectant mother should not do the driving herself.

A certain amount of exercise, in the shape of light housework, may be taken indoors. This is distinctly beneficial if not continued to the point of fatigue, both because of the exercise which it provides, and also the diversion and interest, for these promote mental and physical health. But this indoor exercise must not interfere with, nor to any degree replace the daily exercise which you take out of doors; nor must it include heavy work, such as washing, sweeping, heavy lifting, running a sewing machine by foot or much running up and down stairs.

However, the amount and kind of work which the expectant mother may comfortably and safely do, are so related to what she has been accustomed to, that it is not possible to do more than describe what has proved of benefit for the average woman.

There are women to whom massage and gymnastics are helpful during pregnancy when for some reason the out-of-door activities are not possible or advisable. This might be true of an expectant mother with heart trouble, for example, or of one who is being kept in bed to prevent an abortion and accordingly is a matter which is closely directed by the doctor.

Traveling. In general, traveling is less dangerous for the expectant mother of to-day than formerly because it causes less strain, discomfort and fatigue than in the old days. But the question cannot be settled once for all women nor for all stages of pregnancy. Each woman's general condition must be considered; her tendency to nausea; the length of the journey and the ease with which it may be made; also, whether or not she has ever had or been threatened with an abortion. As a rule, it is considered wise to avoid traveling during the first sixteen and the last four weeks of pregnancy, and at the time of the month when menstruation would ordinarily occur. Certainly a journey should not be undertaken at any time during pregnancy without a doctor's permission.

Rest and Sleep. When we studied the changes that take place during pregnancy we found that as the abdomen increased in size and weight the expectant mother was required to make a constant, though unconscious effort to stand upright. This is probably one reason for the fatigue which she so often feels without apparent cause, and why, upon exertion, she tires more easily than usual.

Accordingly, you may find it necessary to rest frequently during the day in order to avoid the ill effects of fatigue. It is a good plan to work and exercise in short periods rather than long, always lying down when tired, and for an hour or two after the noon meal. You should be careful not to be over active or to overexert yourself at the time when menstruation would occur if you were not pregnant, for fear of bringing on an abortion. This precaution is particularly important during the first four months, the period when abortions occur most frequently.

Since eight hours' sleep is usually considered necessary to keep the average person in good condition, you can scarcely expect to get along satisfactorily with less. In fact, this is so important to your general well-being that you should make a serious effort to secure it.

Fresh air during the day and open windows at night; prudent eating; a comfortable bed furnished with warm but light bedding; warm baths; a hot water bag to the feet and a hot drink upon retiring are all conducive to sleep.

But in addition to these, and perhaps of even more importance, are cheerfulness and a tranquil, untroubled state of mind.

Breasts. Breast feeding is the most urgent single need of the baby, for whose coming we are making preparations, and practically every mother, excepting those with definite physical disability, can supply this need of her baby's if she gives herself proper care both before and after his birth. You will be glad to know in this connection that everything that promotes your general health helps to prepare you to nurse your baby, but there is need also for care of the breasts and nipples themselves, to make the nursing satisfactory, and to prevent sore nipples and possibly even breast abscesses.

Briefly, this local care consists of supporting heavy breasts, but avoiding pressure; bringing out flat or retracted nipples and toughening the skin which covers them.

After they become heavy and uncomfortable the breasts may be supported by brassières, which are snug below the breasts, loose over the breasts themselves and suspended from shoulder straps; or by some such binder as is shown in Fig. 11, which answers the same purpose.

If your nipples are flat or retracted, you should begin about the fifth month to make them more prominent in order that when the baby nurses he may be able to grasp them easily. There are several ways of accomplishing this, all of them in the nature of massage, but whatever is done must be done regularly and persistently. One simple and effective method is to grasp the nipple between the thumb and forefinger, draw it out, hold it for a moment, then release it and allow it to retract. This should be done over and over, two or three times daily. Or the unstoppered opening of a warm bottle may be placed over a flat nipple and held in place until the nipple is drawn up into the neck of the bottle as it cools and a partial vacuum is formed.

The toughening of the nipples should be begun eight weeks before the baby is expected. There are two general methods which seem to give about equally satisfactory results. One is to soften the skin, and the other is to harden it. In either case the nipples should first be scrubbed gently with a soft brush or cloth, warm water and soap, for about five minutes night and morning. After the scrubbing they should be rubbed with lanolin, cocoa butter or vaselin and covered with a piece of clean soft cloth or gauze, to protect the clothing. Or, they may be bathed with a wash consisting of equal parts of a saturated solution of boracic acid and 95 per cent alcohol. You will probably have to have a druggist prepare this for you because of the alcohol.

But no matter which course is followed the care must be regular to be effective. You will find that matters will be simplified if you will assemble in one place and keep in readiness the soap, brush and lotion or ointment which you use each time, using them for no other purpose.

Care of the Teeth. It is very important for the expectant mother to give her teeth scrupulous care from the beginning of pregnancy, for in addition to the ordinary wear and tear with which we all have to cope, her tendency to have an acid stomach makes her mouth acid and this is bad for her teeth. Accordingly, in addition to using dental floss and brushing your teeth after each meal, you should use an alkaline mouth wash several times daily, particularly after vomiting and before retiring, for much damage may be done by the acid secretions in the mouth if they are allowed to bathe the teeth during the long night stretches. Common baking soda (a teaspoonful to a tumbler of water), lime water or milk of magnesia all make excellent mouth washes. It is important, also, that you consult a dentist as soon as you know that you are pregnant and have any necessary repairs done promptly, for delay may be serious.

COMMON DISCOMFORTS DURING PREGNANCY

You may have a number of minor ills and temporary disturbances during pregnancy which are not serious but capable of making you very uncomfortable, and which you may sometimes relieve yourself. But should they be severe or persistent, you should consult your doctor at once. The most common of these minor discomforts may be grouped as digestive disturbances and "pressure symptoms."

Chief among the digestive disturbances are "morning sickness," "heartburn," "distress" and flatulence or "gas."

"**Morning sickness**" is probably the commonest discomfort of pregnancy as it occurs in about half of all cases. Because of the expectant mother's tendency to nausea during the early months, it may be brought on by slight causes which would not produce nausea under ordinary conditions. While it is true that grief, anxiety, fright, shock, incessant worry, fits of temper or brooding may induce nausea when the diet is entirely satisfactory, nausea and even vomiting may be caused in the expectant mother just as they may in any one else by indiscretions in diet, rapid or overeating. On the other hand, simple, light food taken in small quantities, five or six times daily, eaten slowly and masticated thoroughly; the cultivation of a happy frame of mind; exercise and fresh air all tend to prevent this very uncomfortable condition.

Prevention is of great importance, as the habit of vomiting is acquired easily but broken up with difficulty.

When "morning sickness" occurs, however, the sufferer is often relieved by eating two or three hard, unsweetened crackers or crisp toast, immediately upon awaking and then lying still for half or three quarters of an hour. She should then dress slowly, sitting down as much as possible while doing so, and eat her regular breakfast. Lying flat, without a pillow for a little while after meals, or whenever having the slightest feeling of sickness, will frequently prevent, and also relieve nausea. Sometimes comfort is derived from the use of either hot or cold applications over the stomach. Some expectant mothers find that they can prevent nausea by having hot coffee, or even a full breakfast before arising. But the habit of having breakfast in bed should not be cultivated lightly, for in spite of yourself it is likely to make you feel like an invalid, the thing you should carefully avoid. So don't do it unless your doctor orders it.

"Heartburn," so called, which is suffered by so many expectant mothers, has nothing to do with the heart. It is due entirely to too much acid in the stomach and is usually felt as a burning sensation, which starts in the stomach and rises into the throat. It may be prevented, as a rule, by taking a tablespoonful of olive oil or a cupful of cream or rich milk fifteen or twenty minutes before meals and avoiding fat and fried food at the meals themselves. Or, it may be enough simply to avoid eating fats and fatty foods. Since the painful, burning sensation is directly due to too much acid in the stomach, it usually may be relieved by taking a tablespoonful of lime water; a teaspoonful of sodium bicarbonate in water; a small piece of magnesium carbonate; or a drink of any alkaline water that one fancies.

"Distress." Another common discomfort of pregnancy is called "distress" by the sufferers themselves, and occurs after eating. It may be neither heartburn nor pain, but resemble both and make the expectant mother very miserable. It is usually suffered by women who eat rapidly, do not chew their food thoroughly or who eat more at one time than the stomach can hold comfortably. This is one more reason for taking small amounts of food at a time, eating slowly and masticating thoroughly.

Flatulence, or "gas," may or may not be associated with heartburn, but is fairly common among expectant mothers, and is rather uncomfortable. A daily bowel movement is of prime importance in preventing and relieving flatulence and at the same time foods which form gases should be carefully omitted from the diet. The chief offenders are parsnips, beans, corn, fried foods, sweets of all kinds, pastry and very sweet desserts. Yeast cakes and artificially fermented milk sometimes help to prevent flatulence.

Pressure Symptoms. Under the general heading of pressure symptoms are several forms of discomfort resulting from pressure of the enlarged uterus (containing the baby) on the blood-vessels which return from the lower part of the body, thus interfering with the flow of blood back to the heart. The commonest pressure symptoms are swollen feet, varicose veins, hemorrhoids (piles), cramps in the legs and shortness of breath. They may appear at any time during the last half of pregnancy and they grow worse as the weeks wear on.

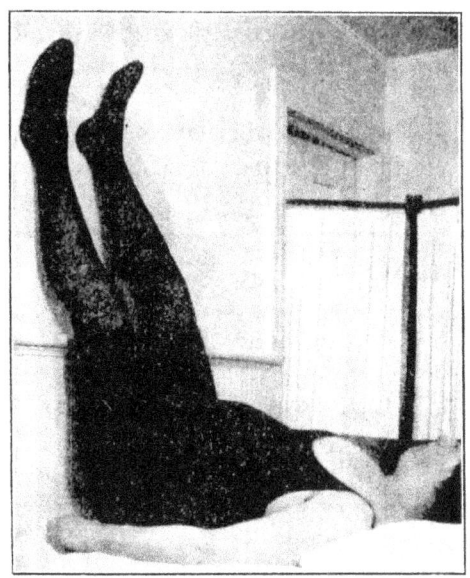

Fig. 14.—Right-angled position to relieve swelling or varicose veins of the feet and legs. (By courtesy of the Maternity Centre Association.)

Swelling of the feet is very common, and when very slight may not be serious or particularly uncomfortable. The swelling may be confined to the back of the ankle, which grows white and shining, or it may extend all the way up the legs to the thighs. Sitting down, with the feet resting on a chair, or lying down with the feet elevated on a pillow will give a certain amount of relief. If the swelling and discomfort are extreme, the expectant mother may have to go to bed until they subside, but very often she will be relieved by elevating her feet or assuming the right-angled position shown in Fig. 14, for even a little while, several times a day. But while employing these harmless measures to make yourself comfortable, you must remember that the swelling of your feet and ankles is one of the symptoms that your doctor wants to know about. For this reason you should promptly report to him even the slightest swelling and begin to measure and save your urine for examination.

Varicose veins are not peculiar to pregnancy but they are among the pressure symptoms which frequently appear during the later months, particularly among women who have borne children. The enlargement of the veins is not usually serious but it may cause a good deal of discomfort. While varicose veins may occur in the vulva, they are usually confined to the legs, and both legs are about equally affected. Sometimes, however, the veins in the right leg are more distended than those in the left, or the right side alone may be affected.

Considerable relief may be obtained by keeping off the feet, particularly by elevating them, and also by the use of elastic bandages. When an expectant mother finds it difficult or nearly impossible to sit or lie down for any length of time, she may secure great relief in a few moments by lying flat on the bed with her legs extended straight into the air, at right angles to her body, resting against the wall or head board, as shown in Fig. 14. This right-angled position for five minutes, three or four times a day, will accomplish wonders in reducing varicose veins.

A spiral elastic bandage, also, will give comfort and help to prevent the veins from growing larger, if applied freshly after each time that the leg is elevated. The most satisfactory bandages, from the standpoint of expense, comfort and cleanliness, are of stockinette or of flannel cut on the bias, measuring three or four inches wide and eight or nine yards long. If made of flannel, the selvages should be whipped together smoothly so that there is neither ridge nor pucker at the seam. The bandage should be wrapped around the leg with firm, even pressure, starting with a few turns over the foot to secure it, and leaving the heel uncovered, carried up the leg to a point above the highest swollen vessels. As a rule the bandage may be left off at night.

There are satisfactory elastic stockings on the market, but they are fairly expensive, often cannot be washed and seem to offer no practical advantage over the bandages.

Swollen veins in the vulva may be relieved by lying flat and elevating the hips, or by lying on the side with the hips elevated on a pillow for a few moments several times a day, as shown in Fig. 15.

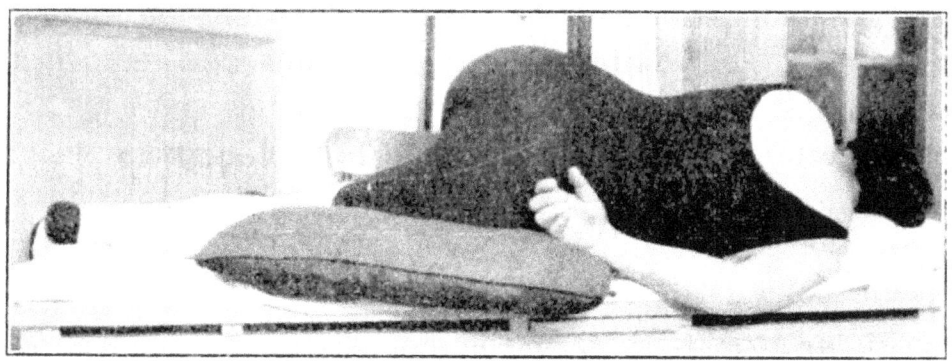

Fig. 15.—Lying on the side with hips elevated to relieve swelling or varicose veins of the vulva. (By courtesy of the Maternity Centre Association.)

Hemorrhoids, or "piles," are virtually varicose veins which protrude from the rectum, but, unlike those in the legs, are extremely painful. As it is the straining in constipation that causes these enlarged veins to protrude from the rectum, this is one more reason for preventing constipation, for a pregnant woman whose bowels move freely every day rarely has hemorrhoids. If hemorrhoids appear, and give pain, the first step is to soften the fingers with vaselin and gently push the hemorrhoids back into the rectum. You can do this quite easily for yourself. You should notify your doctor if you have hemorrhoids, but while waiting to see him, if you are very uncomfortable you will be almost certain to find relief in lying down with your hips elevated on one or two pillows; applying an ice bag to the rectum, or ice-cold cloths or cloths wrung from equal parts of water and witch hazel. Sometimes the hemorrhoids are worse during the first few days after the baby is born but as a rule they disappear when the ultimate cause is removed, which in this case is pressure made by the baby.

Cramps in the legs, numbness or tingling may be caused by pressure of the large, heavy uterus upon nerves supplying the lower extremities. Lying down, applying heat and rubbing the painful parts will usually relieve the discomfort.

Shortness of breath is sometimes very troublesome toward the end of pregnancy, and as may be easily understood, is due to the upward, and not downward pressure of the uterus. For this reason the discomfort is made worse by lying down and relieved by one's sitting up or being well propped up on pillows or a back rest.

Vaginal Discharge. Although the normal vaginal discharge is increased during the later months of pregnancy you should tell your doctor if your discharge is very free. You should not take douches to remove it, unless your doctor orders them, for the normal discharge gives you a certain amount of protection against infection. If it is irritating or causes itching or burning you may obtain relief by avoiding the use of soap and by bathing the uncomfortable parts with water, containing a teaspoonful of sodium bicarbonate to a pint, or with olive oil.

Itching of the skin is a fairly common discomfort, and is possibly a result of irritating material being excreted by the skin glands and deposited upon the surface of the body. The local irritation usually may be relieved, if not very severe, by bathing the uncomfortable areas with the solution of sodium bicarbonate as above, or a lotion consisting of a pint of lime water, half an ounce of glycerin and thirty drops of carbolic acid. It is a good plan, also, to drink more water, in order to promote the activity of the skin, kidneys and bowels, and thus dilute the material that may be responsible for the itching and increase its elimination through all channels.

Some women complain of discomfort caused by the stretching of the skin over the enlarged abdomen. There is a very old belief that rubbing the skin with oil will relieve this sensation and also prevent the appearance of the purplish streaks described in a previous chapter. There seems to be little foundation for this belief, but if a woman fancies that she is safer and more comfortable after oiling her abdomen, there is certainly no reason why she should not do so.

HELPING TO PREVENT COMPLICATIONS

I have described to you the details of personal hygiene which your doctor is likely to want you to adopt during your months of expectancy, and some of the simple things that you may do to relieve minor discomforts when they arise, for having these things in black and white may make the whole matter a little easier for you.

But there is still more that you can do to help the doctor help you. You can tell him about any discomfort or any new condition that appears, and follow his advice instead of talking it over with your family or friends. This will make it possible for him to prevent serious complications by treating them in the very beginning.

You have probably learned, in one way or another, that the complications associated with childbirth that are most serious are infections (childbed fever), convulsions, abortions or miscarriages and severe bleeding, but perhaps you have not heard that you, yourself, can help greatly in the prevention of all of these conditions, in your own case, and chiefly by little more than exercising good common sense.

Your part in preventing childbed fever, if your baby is to be born at home, lies in having in readiness a clean room, sterile sheets, towels, gauze pads, etc., as will be described in the next chapter.

Concerning the other complications we shall say a word here.

Convulsions. You can do a great deal toward preventing the condition that causes convulsions by following the advice about your personal care that we have just gone over and by making it possible for the doctor to treat early symptoms promptly. In fact, after looking over the records of many thousands of mothers who have had prenatal care, it seems almost safe to say that the expectant mother who follows such a course will not have convulsions.

One of the commonest of the early symptoms is headache, sometimes persistent and very severe. Others which you can detect are blurred vision, spots before the eyes, dizziness, vomiting which is more persistent or severe than could be called "morning sickness," puffiness under the eyes or elsewhere about the face or hands, swelling of the feet and ankles and severe pain in the stomach. It might be that if you had even one of these symptoms your doctor would think it worth while to put you to bed and give you nothing but milk, or only water, for a day or two, not because you were sick, but to keep you from being so, on the same principle that you darn a thin place in a stocking to keep a hole from coming.

In any event, tell your doctor about the symptoms and let him decide what is to be done, for therein lies your safety.

Miscarriages. The question of abortions, miscarriages and premature births is one of enormous importance, and one about which there is a good deal of misunderstanding. As to the meaning of the terms, many women are puzzled to know the difference between them. Doctors are not likely to use the word miscarriage, but will describe as an abortion a termination of pregnancy which occurs before the end of the seventh month and as premature labors those occurring from that time until the expected date of confinement. In the minds of lay people, however, the term abortion is often associated with criminal practice, miscarriage being a term loosely applied to all births occurring before the seventh month, while the premature baby is the one born after the seventh month of pregnancy but before the expected date of confinement.

Of all of these accidents, abortions are the most frequent, though in the nature of things it is impossible to say how often they occur. They sometimes happen so early in pregnancy that the expectant mother is unaware of the accident; or if she does know of it she may make the mistake of taking no notice of it or regard it of so little consequence that she does not consult a doctor. But such information as is available suggests that at least one out of every five pregnancies ends in abortion, the tragedy of this being that it is very largely a preventable disaster.

Since the ovum is insecurely attached to the uterine lining until the sixteenth or eighteenth week, an abortion is more likely to occur during this time than later, while of this period, the second and third months seem to be the most perilous. Abortions are less likely to happen during first pregnancies than succeeding ones and their frequency seems to increase with the number of pregnancies. They occur more often among women over thirty-five years than in younger ones, and in all cases are most likely to take place at the time when menstruation would fall due were the woman not pregnant.

The prevention of abortions is of such obvious importance and there is so much that you can do to this end, that we shall take up the question somewhat at length. Preventive treatment really begins very early. In the discussion about menstruation we referred to the importance of finding out the cause of painful periods, in the interest of good obstetrics, since inflammation of the uterine lining or a misplaced uterus might be responsible for the pain and if neglected might cause an abortion later on. The correction of such troubles, no matter when they are discovered, is an early step toward preventing abortions.

But after pregnancy has actually begun, there are certain preventive measures which have proved to be very effective. A woman who is pregnant for the first time, and who, therefore, does not know whether she is likely to have an abortion or not, should avoid such risks as fatigue, sweeping, lifting or moving heavy objects, running a sewing machine by foot, running, jumping, dancing, traveling or any action which might jar or jolt her during the first sixteen or eighteen weeks.

An expectant mother who has had an abortion will have to take even greater precautions, as she is in more danger than is a woman who has not had this experience. It is of prime importance, to begin with, that she have the cause of her previous abortion discovered, and if possible corrected. And since the accident is most likely to be repeated at about the same time, or a little earlier, in each succeeding pregnancy it is a wise precaution for the expectant mother to remain quietly in bed for at least a week before and after the time when an abortion may be feared.

Complete rest and relaxation are such effective preventive measures that patients with a tendency to have abortions who have been willing to stay in bed during most of their pregnancy have sometimes been rewarded by going through the entire period and in the end giving birth to a normal, fully developed baby. As out-of-door exercise is clearly impossible in such cases, it is important that the patient keep her room very well ventilated all of the time, and possibly, under the doctor's direction, have massage or bed exercises.

The marital relation is usually considered inadvisable in all cases after the eighth month of pregnancy, and among women who have had abortions or miscarriages it is best omitted throughout the entire period. This is particularly true of women over thirty-five who are pregnant for the first time.

To sum it up in a word, your part in preventing an abortion or miscarriage after pregnancy has begun, consists largely of avoiding fatigue; resting when tired; avoiding physical shocks such as blows upon the abdomen, jolts or falls particularly during the first sixteen or eighteen weeks and at the time when menstruation would ordinarily occur if you were not pregnant, and avoiding overwork during the later weeks of pregnancy.

The common symptoms of abortions or miscarriages are bleeding, often accompanied by recurring pain, beginning in the small of the back and finally felt as cramps in the lower part of the abdomen. Since menstruation is suspended during pregnancy you should always regard bleeding or a bloody discharge as a symptom of a possible miscarriage, whether you have pain or not. Upon its appearance you should send for the doctor, go to bed at once and keep absolutely quiet.

Should you be so unfortunate as to have a miscarriage, in spite of all your precautions, bear in mind that you will need to stay in bed quite as long afterwards and have the same care as though you had given birth to a fully developed baby. It is because so many women fail to appreciate this that abortions and premature births are often followed by ill health and invalidism. Under proper care, an abortion or premature labor is not, of itself, any more serious for a woman than a normal delivery.

Bleeding from the vagina, or a sudden increase in the size of the abdomen with perspiration and a sudden feeling of faintness, may be the beginning of severe bleeding, or hemorrhage, from any one of a number of causes, and in such a case the expectant mother should notify her doctor, go to bed at once and keep quiet until he arrives.

Summing up the whole question of preventing complications, we find that the following symptoms may be forerunners of serious trouble and therefore should be watched for and reported to the doctor as soon as they are noticed:

1. Persistent or severe vomiting.
2. Persistent or severe headache.
3. Dizziness.

4. Blurred vision or the appearance of black spots before the eyes.

5. Puffiness under the eyes, or elsewhere about the face.

6. Swelling of the feet, ankles or hands.

7. Sharp pains, particularly in the stomach.

8. Prolonged failure to feel the baby's movements after they have once been felt.

9. Bleeding, or a bloody discharge.

10. Pain in the small of the back followed by cramp-like pains in the abdomen, before the expected date of confinement.

11. Unwarranted mental depression, anxiety or apprehension.

These are generally accepted as the danger signs of pregnancy, any one of which, alone or in combination with one or more of the others, is of importance. In addition to these it really is important that you talk to your doctor or your nurse freely if you are feeling worried or depressed about anything at all. Sometimes one feels blue without knowing why, and if you should feel so during your pregnancy you should not keep it to yourself but talk it over with your doctor or your nurse.

When all is said and done, what we want for each expectant mother is little more than that she shall live a normal, regular, wholesome life; that she shall be able, and what is of equal importance, be willing to weave into her everyday life the principles of personal care which every one should adopt; that she shall watch and be watched for symptoms of complications throughout the entire period of pregnancy, in order that they may be detected early, speedily treated and serious troubles thereby prevented.

The adoption of such simple precautions will pave the highroad to health and happiness for yourself and your baby.

CHAPTER VI
MAKING READY FOR THE BABY

In making ready for the actual arrival of the baby there are several factors to consider, chief among them being the doctor; the nurse; the place where the baby is to be born; the room he is to occupy and an equipment which will facilitate the care of yourself and the baby, at the time of his birth and afterwards.

Of course you have long since placed yourself under a doctor's care, so that is settled. If you are in the care of a privately engaged physician, he will, in all probability tell you his wishes in regard to your engaging a nurse. She should be satisfactory to both you and the doctor from the standpoint of training and professional fitness as well as her personality. The selection of the nurse, therefore, should be made in coöperation with your doctor. It is wise to engage her during the early part of your pregnancy both to insure your securing the one that you and the doctor want especially, and to have that much of the preparation off your mind. It is usually a good plan to engage the nurse to hold herself in readiness to respond to your call at any time after two weeks before the expected date of your confinement. Quite reasonably, if she is obliged to give up or refuse an engagement in order to hold herself available for you, from a given date, she will do so at your expense. Try to arrange to have the nurse stay with you for six weeks after the baby is born, even though this involves considerable financial sacrifice on your part. Of course if you can afford to keep her still longer, so much the better.

All of this is in case you are in the care of a privately engaged physician and are to have a special nurse. If you are being cared for during pregnancy by doctors and nurses connected with a dispensary, health center or prenatal clinic, they will advise with you about your nursing care at the time of confinement and afterwards.

The next question to consider is whether the baby is to be born at your home or in a hospital. The doctor who is advising you will have his wishes on this subject, too, and as they are entirely in your interest, you will, of course, do as he advises. You will be likely to find that for the birth of the first baby he will want you to go to a hospital, if there is a good one available; also if you have had any symptoms of complications during this pregnancy or difficulty with previous labors.

If you are going to a hospital you or your doctor will make the necessary arrangements about your room, well in advance of the date upon which you expect to go, in order to feel sure that a room will be ready for you.

It sometimes happens, that for a variety of reasons it is nearly or quite impossible for the expectant mother to go to a hospital, or that her doctor is entirely willing that she shall be confined at home. If it is decided that you are to remain at home, it will be possible, with a little planning and effort on your part, to imitate very nearly in your own home the advantages which are offered by a hospital.

You will remember that in the last chapter I mentioned childbed fever as being one of the serious complications, associated with childbirth, that could be prevented by careful work. In the old days, when the importance of cleanliness was not appreciated, this fever was very common in maternity hospitals, but nowadays it seldom occurs in well conducted institutions because the doctors and nurses know how to do clean work and also because they have clean things to work with. So if you are to be attended at home by a good doctor and a good nurse you may make the conditions of your confinement practically ideal by providing a clean room and such an outfit of sterile sheets, towels, dressings and certain other articles as would be available for their use in a hospital.

Suppose we settle the question of the rooms first.

It is a very important one but need not be the bugbear that some people think it is. In all probability you will have no choice as to a room for yourself and will have to use the one you ordinarily occupy. Should you have a choice, however, it will be well to select one that is cool and shady, if the baby is coming during the summer, but one that is bright and sunny for occupancy during most of the year. It should be conveniently near a bathroom, if possible; have an adjoining room for the nurse and one near by for the baby.

The ideal to work toward is: A room with a washable floor with small, light rugs; freshly laundered curtains at the windows but no heavy draperies; a single brass or iron bedstead, about thirty inches high, with a firm mattress, and so placed as to be accessible from both sides and with the foot in a good light, either by day or night; a bedside table and two others (folding card tables are a great convenience); a bureau; a washstand, unless there is a bathroom on the same floor; one or two comfortable chairs, two or three straight chairs and a couch or *chaise longue*, all of which should be of wood or wicker or covered with freshly laundered chintzes.

Between such a room as this and the one that must be used there may be a wide difference, but it will be worth while to approach this standard as nearly as possible. It is not necessary to make the room bare; in fact, it should be as cheerful and pretty as is compatible with cleanliness. There is no objection to pictures on the walls, but the room should be free from useless, small articles which are likely to be dust catchers, give the nurse unnecessary work and occupy space needed for other things.

The room should be given a thorough house-cleaning about two weeks before the baby is expected. If there is a carpet on the floor that cannot be taken up conveniently, it might be well to have in readiness a large canvas or rubber or an abundance of newspapers to protect the floor near the bed. If the bed is low, the attentions of the doctor and nurse will be made much easier if you have ready four solid blocks of wood, of the same size, upon which to elevate the bed, after the casters have been removed. The blocks should be of such a size as to bring the height of the bed up to thirty inches. And it is important, too, to have a large board, or table leaves, at hand, to slip under the mattress to make it firm, particularly if the bed is soft or sinks in the middle.

The chief requisites for the baby's room are that it may be well ventilated and easily cleaned. The floor should be of hard wood, or covered with linoleum, in order that it may be wiped up with a damp cloth every day, and the walls should be freshly papered, or, better still, painted. As bright light and glare are bad for the baby the walls would better be of a soft shade, such as grayish green or blue, than white, and there should be dark shades at the windows, in order that the room may be darkened at will.

The furnishings may consist of a brass or enameled crib, with a hair mattress; a chest of drawers; a low straight chair and low rocker, both without arms, and a low table for the baby's toilet articles. An ordinary kitchen table, enameled and with the legs sawed off, serves admirably. All of the furniture should have smooth, washable surfaces, such as hard wood or enamel, and the walls should be free from pictures, for the baby's room will have to be kept scrupulously clean and free from dust.

So much for the rooms.

When it comes to the question of providing the outfit to be used in your personal care, the matter of nightgowns and the like will be determined by your tastes and your means, rather than by specific needs. But six or eight nightgowns, a warm bed jacket if the weather is cool, a dressing-gown and a pair of slippers, will probably be enough to keep you fresh and comfortable, so far as these things are concerned, whether you are in a hospital or at home.

But the preparation of necessary dressings and other articles for a home confinement is a different matter and you should learn the wishes of your doctor concerning them.

If his instructions are not specific, you may find that the following lists will be helpful guides in assembling an equipment which will prove adequate to meet the ordinary requirements of a home confinement. Most of the articles listed, or satisfactory substitutes, are to be found in the average household, but they should be gotten together in one place so as to be ready at a moment's notice.

For the Confinement and Your Own Care:

Plenty of sheets, pillow cases and towels.
4 sanitary belts.
1 piece rubber sheeting or oil cloth, $1 \times 1½$ yards.
1 piece rubber sheeting or oilcloth, $2 \times 1½$ yards.
Two or three dozen safety-pins.
Hot water bag with flannel cover.
1 two-quart fountain syringe.
1 douche pan.
1 bed-pan.

2 covered slop jars or covered pails.
3 basins, about 16, 14 and 12 inches in diameter.
2 stiff nail brushes, nail scissors and file or orange stick.
3 agate or enamel pitchers, holding at least 1 quart each.
Medicine glass.
Medicine dropper.
2 bent glass drinking tubes.
100 bichlorid tablets.
4 ounces chloroform.
4 ounces boric acid powder.
4 ounces green soap.
1 pint grain alcohol.
Small jar of vaselin to be sterilized.
Lard, olive oil, vaselin or albolene to oil the baby.
Roll of adhesive plaster, 1 inch wide.
One package of absorbent cotton.
One clinical thermometer.

In addition to these, a certain supply of sterile dressings will be needed. Complete outfits of such dressings, sterilized and ready for use, may be obtained from any one of a number of firms, of which your doctor will know; or they may be prepared by the nurse, or you yourself may prepare and sterilize the following:

One dozen towels.

Three sheets. Five or six dozen sanitary pads, about 10 inches long and 4 inches wide, made of gauze and cotton batting with a top layer of absorbent cotton.

Two to four bed pads, about 30 inches square and 4 inches thick, made of gauze and cotton waste or cotton batting with a top layer of absorbent cotton; or of newspapers covered with muslin.

One pair of leggings made of canton- or outing-flannel, either loose fitting hose reaching to the thighs or a yard square folded diagonally and stitched on one side. See Fig. 16. Five or six dozen gauze sponges, made by folding pieces of gauze 18 inches square into small pads with all raw edges inside.

Two or three dozen gauze squares, 4 inches square.

Four or five dozen cotton pledgets, or wads of absorbent cotton about the size of an egg with the edges drawn together between thumb and finger and twisted into a spiral.

Six pieces of bobbin or narrow tape, 9 inches long, to tie the baby's cord.

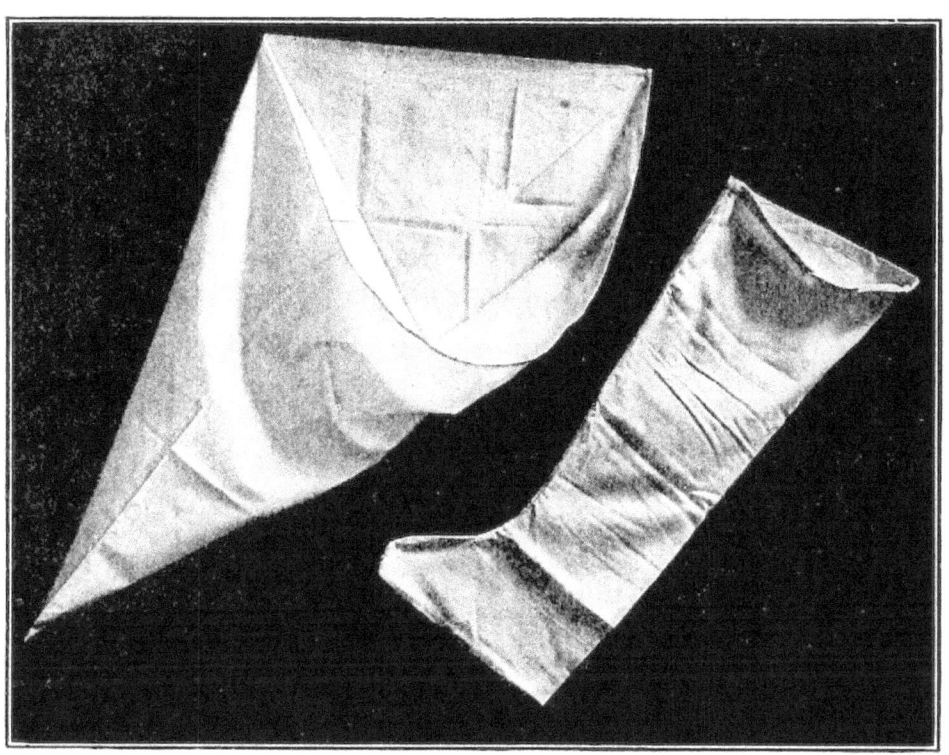

Fig. 16.—Two types of easily made leggings, suitable for use at the baby's birth.

To make these supplies you will need about four pounds of absorbent cotton, 6 or 8 packages of cotton batting, and possibly 40 yards of gauze in addition to cotton flannel for the hose.

In preparing the dressings for sterilization, you may divide them into packages as follows: The sheets in one package; 6 towels in a package; 6 sanitary pads in a package; 2 delivery pads in a package; the gauze squares in two packages; the leggings in one package; the bobbin in one package. The sponges and pledgets should be put up in bags or small pillow cases, 2 or 3 dozen in a bag. Wrap each package in heavy muslin, either new or old, using pieces large enough to well protect the contents from contamination by dust or handling, tie them securely with string and sterilize as follows:

Fill a wash boiler about a quarter full of water and fashion a hammock by securely tying a towel or strip of muslin to the handles at each end and allowing it to hang so that the bottom of the hammock is about halfway down in the boiler. As the weight of the dressings makes the hammock sag low in the middle it is a wise precaution to place a rack or support of some kind in the bottom of the boiler, to hold the dressings well above the bubbling water, at the point where they hang lowest. Pile the dressings into the hammock, cover the boiler tightly and keep the water boiling vigorously for an hour; dry the packages in the sun, or by placing them in the oven for a few moments, taking care that they are not loosened or opened, and at the end of twenty-four hours repeat the steaming and drying process, wrap the packages in a clean sheet and put them in a drawer or covered box where they may remain undisturbed until needed. The nail brushes, douche pan and fountain syringe may be wrapped in muslin and sterilized in the same way, or the nurse may boil them when the time comes to use them.

Bed pads made of newspapers offer excellent protection and are, of course, less expensive than those made of cotton. They consist of six or eight thicknesses of newspaper opened out to the full size of the page and covered with a piece of freshly laundered muslin which is folded over the edges and basted in place or held with safety-pins, as shown in Fig. 17. These pads may be made virtually sterile by ironing them on the muslin side with a very hot iron, folding the ironed surface inside without touching it, ironing the outside after it is folded and wrapping the pads in a clean sheet or muslin, also recently ironed, and putting them away with the other dressings, in a place protected from dust.

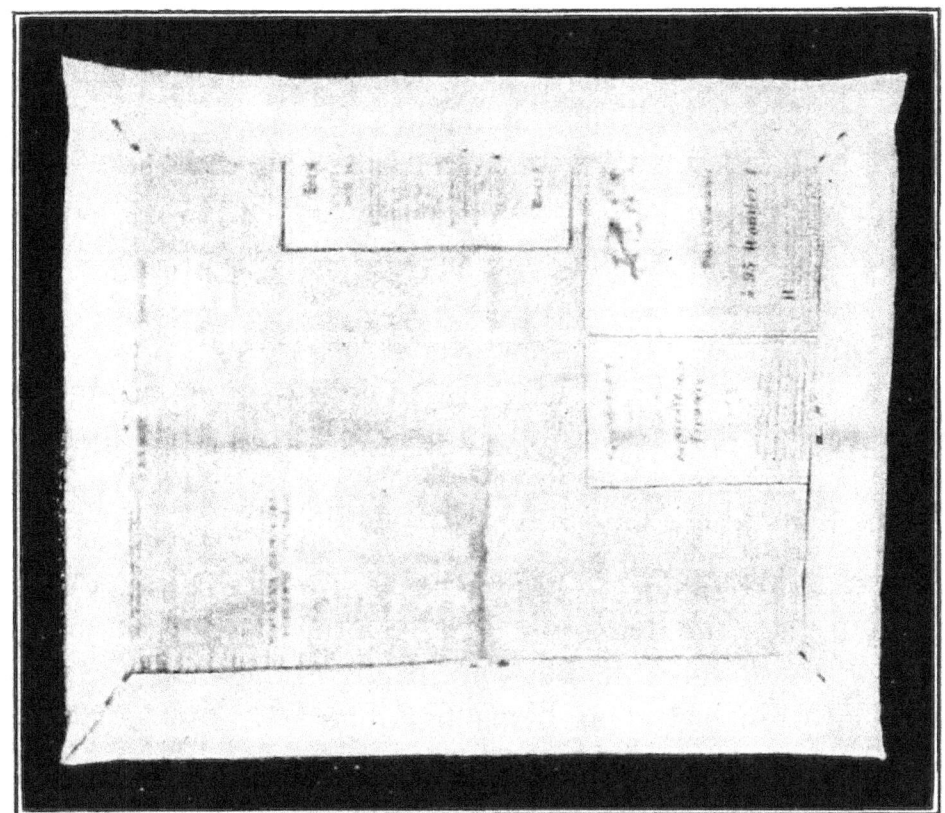

FIG. 17.—Reverse side of pad made of newspapers and old muslin to protect bed during a home confinement. If muslin is held in place with safety-pins it may be removed easily, washed and used for another pad. (By courtesy of the Maternity Centre Association.)

Baby Clothes. In planning the baby clothes, there are a few general principles to bear in mind that are of considerable importance to the baby's welfare. His health actually may be injured by having his clothes too warm or not warm enough, and also if they are tight enough to bind or constrict any part of his body or so ample as to form bunches and wrinkles which will make him uncomfortable and restless.

To be entirely satisfactory his clothes should be simple in design and so made as to slip on easily, fit loosely and at the same time smoothly; the materials should be soft, light and porous. Complete outfits of baby clothes may be bought outright, but few expectant mothers are willing to forego the sheer ecstasy of fashioning the little garments themselves, while they dream dreams of the baby who is to wear them. The following list of garments will meet the baby's needs, and those which you may make are really very simple:

Two to four dozen diapers, about 18 inches square.
Three flannel bands 6 inches wide and 27 inches long, unhemmed.
Three knitted bands with shoulder straps.
Three shirts, infants', size 2, of cotton and wool, silk and wool but not all wool.
Four wool and cotton flannel petticoats.
Four wool and cotton flannel nightgowns.
Six thin white cotton slips, or dresses.
Flannel wrapper or a yard square of flannel for extra wrap in cool room.
Cloak and cap or other wrap for out door use in cool weather.

Let us take these up in turn.

The **diapers** may be of any soft, absorbent, loosely woven material, such as cheesecloth, stockinette, bird's-eye, cotton flannel or thin Turkish toweling, single or double thickness, according to the weight of the material used, and about 18 inches square when hemmed.

The first **bands** are of cotton and wool flannel, torn-straight across the width of the material in 6–inch strips and left unhemmed. After the cord separates, this band is usually replaced by a knitted band with shoulder straps.

The **shirts** should have high necks and long sleeves, come well down over the hips and open all the way down the front. They should be of cotton and wool or silk and wool but not all wool as this is too warm. During very warm weather the shirts should be of thin cotton or silk. It is better to start with size 2 as the smaller size will soon be outgrown.

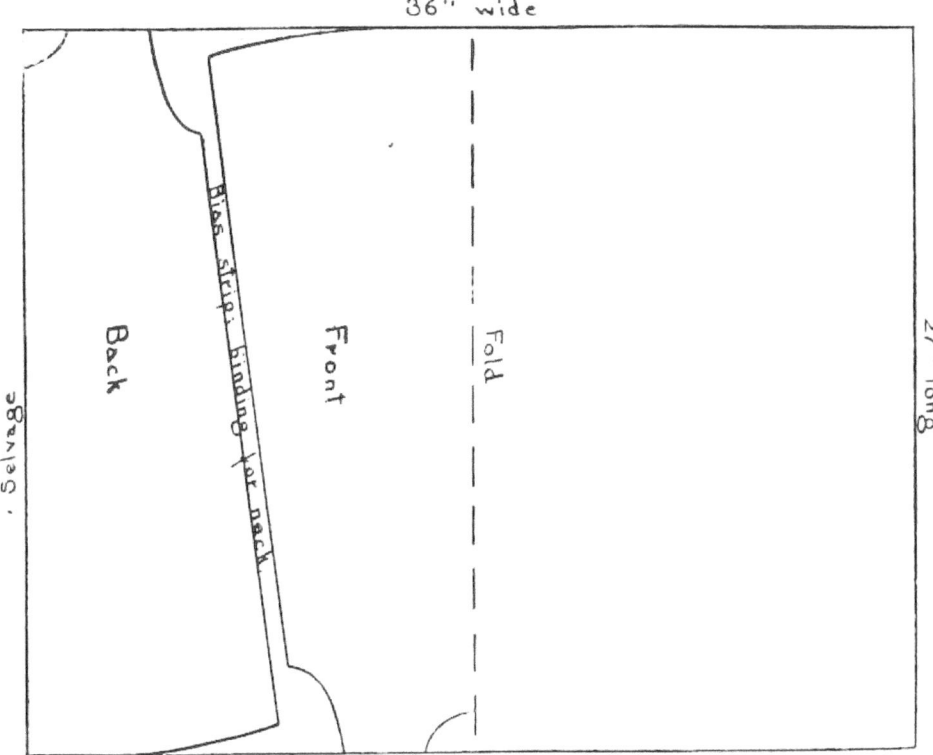

Fig. 18.—Pattern for baby's petticoat (shown in *C*. Fig. 20) requiring ¾ yard of material one yard wide. The cotton dress (*A*) and flannel nightgown (*B*) in Fig. 20, may be made from this pattern with the addition of straight sleeves.

The **petticoat** is a very important item in the baby's wardrobe, for, helping as it does to keep his body evenly warm, it is worn constantly except during very warm weather. It should be a straight little slip, about 27 inches long, hanging from the shoulders, made entirely of flannel, without the broad cotton waistband that has tortured so many babies in days gone by.

The chief purpose of the **dresses** or slips is to keep the petticoats clean and add to the daintiness of the baby's attire and they are made, therefore, of very thin, soft cotton or linen material. They are made from the same pattern as the petticoats, except that they have sleeves and these may be set in or cut out in one piece with the rest of the garment like kimono sleeves, as in Fig. 19.

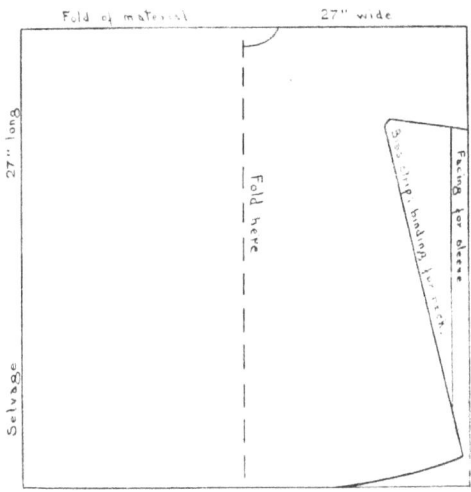

FIG. 19—Pattern for kimono-style dress or nightgown, shown in E, Fig. 20, and requiring 1½ yards of material 27 inches wide.

The **nightgowns** are made like the slips, but of the same part wool flannel as that used for the petticoats.

The petticoats, slips and nightgowns should all open down the back and may be fastened with either tapes or buttons and buttonholes. These fastenings present about equal advantages but there is perhaps a slight preference for buttons as babies sometimes tangle their fingers in tapes or get them in their mouths.

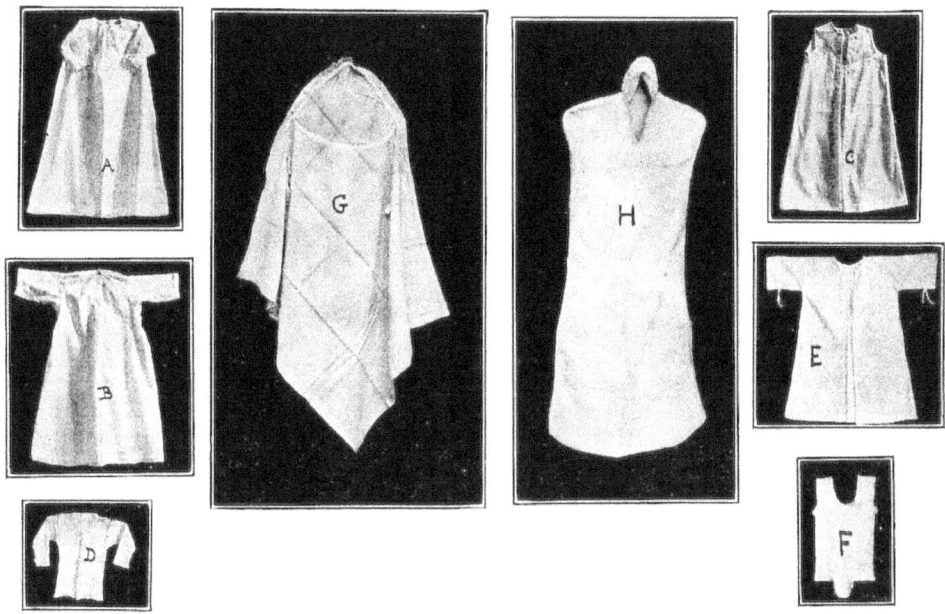

Fig. 20.—An outfit of satisfactory baby clothes:

A. Thin cotton dress, open down the back.
B. Flannel nightgown with set-in-sleeves.
C. "Gertrude" petticoat, open down the back.
D. Shirt, opened all the way down the front.
E. Flannel nightgown with kimono sleeves.
F. Knitted band with shoulder straps.
G. Flannel square with tapes run through casings to form hood of one corner.
H. Bag, with hood, suitable for premature baby or for outdoor sleeping.

A satisfactory little **wrap** to use at first may be made from a yard square of soft, warm material with a hood formed of one corner by running tapes through casings.

Patterns for these baby clothes may be obtained from two or three of the large pattern concerns, or you may cut them out, yourself, by using Figs. 18 and 19 as guides, while Fig. 20 shows how the various little garments look when finished.

The question of **socks** for the new baby is one upon which doctors hold different opinions, some believing that the warmth provided by the petticoat is sufficient; others, that there is an advantage in the extra protection afforded by socks, so you would better learn the wishes of your own doctor in this connection.

Additional Articles Which Are Needed or Useful in the Care of the Baby:

Bath tub, tin, enamel, agate or rubber.
Drying frames for shirts and stockings.
Rubber bath apron.
Flannel, or Turkish toweling bath apron.
Low chair without arms.
Low table.
Screen to protect baby during bath.
Rack upon which to hang clothes to warm during bath.
Scales, with beam and basket or scoop, not the spring variety.
Hot water bag and cover.
Crib, basket or box, to be used as bed.
Folded felt pad, blanket or hair pillow for mattress.
Rubber or oilcloth to cover mattress.
6 crib sheets.
1 thermometer.
2 crib blankets.
Soft towels and wash cloths.
An old blanket to be used for bath blanket.
3 or 4 dozen safety-pins, assorted sizes.
Castile soap.
Boric acid powder.
Olive oil or albolene.
Absorbent cotton pledgets, preferably sterile.
Enamel pail and cover.

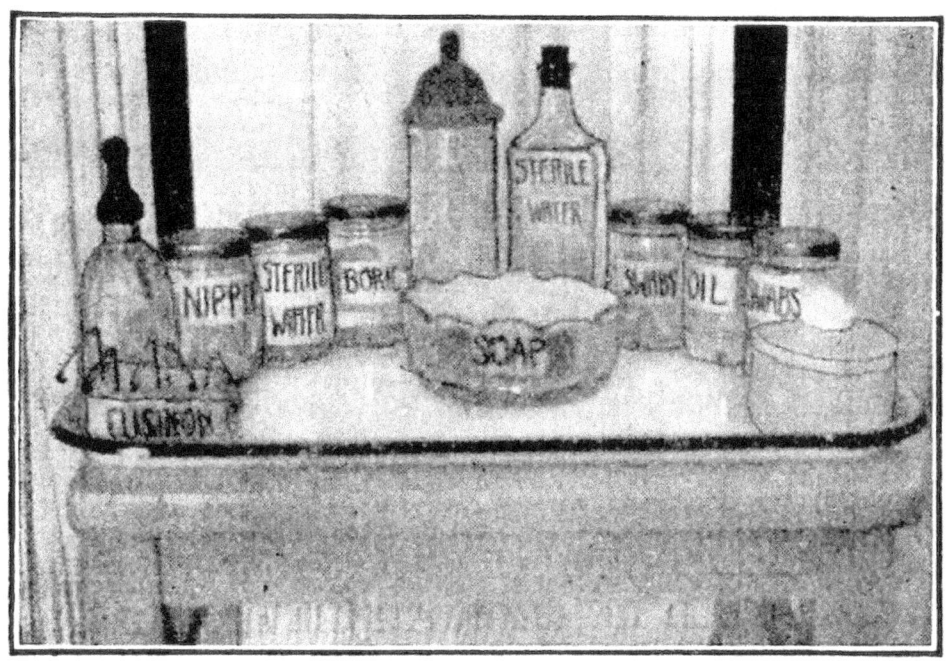

FIG. 21.—Baby's toilet tray equipped with jelly glasses, bottles, celluloid hair receiver for cotton, and a soap dish, as follows:

1. Safety-pins sticking in cake of soap.
2. Jar for sterile nipples.
3. Jar of sterile water.
4. Jar of boracic acid solution.
5. Nursing bottle.
6. Sterile water to drink.
7. Nursing bottle for water.
8. Small tooth pick swabs.
9. Liquid petrolatum.
10. Gauze mouth swabs.
11. Absorbent cotton.
12. Soap.

(By courtesy of the Maternity Centre Association.)

The giving of the baby's daily bath, after he comes, will be greatly simplified if you will assemble beforehand and keep in readiness on a tray or small table, all of the things which are to be used each time. Dainty little outfits for this purpose may be bought, or you may arrange an entirely satisfactory one from jars and bottles to be found in the house, as suggested in Fig. 21.

The above lists of dressings and articles to be used in the care of both mother and baby can be considerably modified, according to one's tastes and means, and still be satisfactory. They merely represent a fair average of what has been found adequate to meet the usual needs of the mother and baby at home.

It will be a good plan for you to have in readiness, by about the end of the seventh calendar month, all of the dressings and other articles to be used during the confinement. This is in case you should have a premature labor, for which the same dressings are needed as in a normal delivery. The baby's clothes, however, will be in time if they are ready by the end of the eighth month. A baby born before this time would probably be so frail that he would be wrapped in cotton at first, instead of being dressed in the clothes ordinarily prepared for a fully developed baby.

If you will make such preparations for the baby's arrival as I have suggested, you will be doing a great deal toward securing his safety and well-being, as well as your own.

CHAPTER VII
THE BABY'S ARRIVAL

During the past nine months you have had the happiness of guarding the little life within you and of making soft, warm garments to have in readiness for the baby when he comes. You have prepared your room and his; folded up the packages of gauze and cotton and prepared all sorts of other things to be pressed into service upon the baby's arrival, and through it all you have dreamed and planned and built the loveliest of castles in Spain.

And now, at last, the baby is coming!

It almost takes your breath away to realize it after all those months of waiting and dreaming, and though it scarcely seems possible, the waiting is almost over.

This same waiting grows very hard toward the end for you are tense with expectation and suspense. The hours and days seem endlessly long, as they pass without giving the looked-for signs that the baby has started. You find it very hard not to grow discouraged and impatient, he seems so long in coming. Your physical discomfort is aggravated by the greater pressure made by the baby during this period, and you cannot get away from it day or night. The desire to urinate is almost constant; your back aches; your feet feel heavy and swollen and the baby disturbs your nights by his increasingly vigorous kicking.

But this does not last long, so try to minimize the fatiguing effects of it all by resting and sleeping as much as possible during the day. The time does slip by and the baby really does come and you don't want to be tired before the big event.

The miracle of the baby's origin at the moment of conception; of his growth and the development of the intricate parts of his little body, is equaled only by the miracle of his birth—his separating from your protecting body and coming into the world as a new human being when the time comes that he is able to exist separately and independently.

Since very early in pregnancy, you will remember, your uterus has been growing alternately hard and soft as the muscles have contracted and relaxed. But these contractions have been as painless, and so far as we know, as fruitless as the contractions of a boy's biceps as he clenches his fist and produces a hard lump on his arm.

But when the baby is ready to take up his life among the rest of us human beings, the contractions of your uterine muscles are altered in such a manner that you gradually become conscious of them and they become so purposeful that they are able slowly but steadily to force the baby down through that narrow part of the pelvis called the inlet, through the cervix, and finally out into the world.

Since, at the proper time you will be able to help these altered muscular contractions to accomplish their high purpose, you will want to watch their progress, with your mind's eye, as far as possible.

Recall, for a moment, the fact that the baby is contained in a sac of fluid in the cavity of the uterus, above the cervix; that the cervix, below, is a canal drawn in tightly at the upper end, or internal os, and also at the lower end, or external os.

Quite evidently after the baby's head has been squeezed through the pelvic inlet by pressure of the uterine contractions, the cervix must open widely in order that he may pass through it, too. And so Nature gradually stretches this narrow canal by using the lowermost part of the bag of waters as a water-wedge and forcing it down into the internal os, a little farther with each pain. The opening grows wider and wider as the bag of waters is pressed farther and farther down into the cervical canal, which also widens slowly, and finally the external os, too, is stretched wide open by the water-wedge. Fig. 22 shows how the cervix looks with the bag of waters pressed against the upper opening and how the entire canal is gradually dilated by this wedge, as it is pressed downward.

As you doubtless know, the process of your baby's emergence into the world and separation from your body is termed **labor**. The onset of labor is usually marked by the expectant mother becoming conscious of the uterine contractions through dragging pains which are felt first in the small of the back and then in the lower part of the abdomen and thighs. In the beginning the pains are feeble and infrequent, but they gradually grow more severe and more frequent. Sometimes the first sign of labor is a gush of fluid, caused by the rupture of the membranes, or the appearance of blood, but these are not typical. Intestinal colic is sometimes mistaken for labor pains by women who are pregnant for the first time, but when the cramps come regularly and the uterus is felt, through the abdominal wall, to grow hard as the pain increases, and soft as it subsides, there can be no doubt that they are labor pains.

This is the time, usually, when you will go to the hospital, if your baby is to be born there, or when you will notify your doctor that you think you are in labor. If you are to remain at home the doctor may want you to send for the nurse at once, in which case he depends upon her to communicate with him. Or he may prefer that you notify him and let him send the nurse. Either arrangement is simple and easy to carry out, but you must be sure that you understand just what the doctor wants you to do when you think labor has started. It is not a bad plan to write down his instructions about this, with the telephone number and street address of the one to be summoned, so that you will know exactly how to proceed when the time comes.

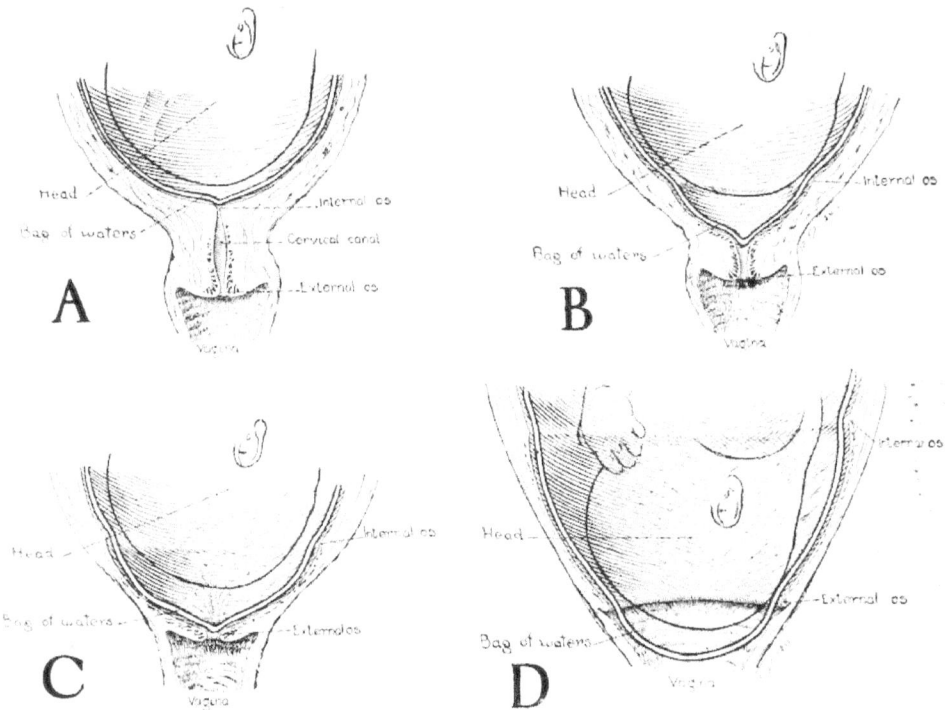

Fig. 22.—Diagrams showing how the cervix is dilated as the bag of waters is forced downward by the uterine contractions.

The entire duration of labor may vary from a few moments to several days, but the average length of the first labor is about eighteen hours and of subsequent births about twelve hours. The process is usually described as being divided into the first, second and third stages of labor, approximately as follows:

	First stage	*Second stage*	*Third stage*	*Total*
First labor	16 hours	1¾ hours	15 minutes	18 hours
Later labors	11 hours	45 minutes	15 minutes	12 hours

The first stage begins with the onset of labor and lasts until the cervical canal is completely dilated; the second stage begins when the cervix is dilated and lasts until the baby is born; the third stage begins with the birth of the baby and lasts until the afterbirth is expelled.

First Stage. The pains are mild at first and occur at intervals of from fifteen to thirty minutes, but they gradually increase in frequency and intensity until by the end of fourteen to sixteen hours, they are very severe, and recur every three or four minutes, each pain lasting about one minute.

The pains begin in the back, then pass slowly forward to the abdomen and down into the thighs.

The average woman is entirely comfortable between pains and until they become very frequent she will usually prefer to be up and about, but if she is on her feet when a contraction begins she will usually seek relief by leaning forward on something secure, as the foot of the bed or a table, or by sitting down until the pain subsides. As time passes, there is an increasing, sometimes persistent desire to empty the bowels and bladder because of pressure upon these two organs by the baby's head as it is forced slowly downward. There may be vomiting, also when the cervix becomes nearly, or quite dilated.

In the course of the stretching process, the cervix sustains many tiny tears from which blood oozes and tinges the vaginal discharge. This bloodstained discharge is often called the "show" and usually appears toward the end of the first stage.

When the cervix is fully dilated, the membranes, or bag of waters, usually rupture, and there is a sudden gush of fluid, but the rupture of the membranes does not necessarily mark the end of the first stage. Sometimes, though not often, they break before labor begins, thus producing what is known as a "dry" labor. They may rupture before the cervix is fully dilated or they may not rupture at all until the doctor punctures them to facilitate the baby's birth.

If the nurse is delayed in reaching you, there is a good deal that you can do and have done, during this first stage of labor, in the way of preparing for the baby's arrival, this preparation relating in general to yourself and to the room including placement of the sterile dressings.

As to yourself, try first to picture what takes place during the fifteen or sixteen hours of the first stage. The baby's head has usually passed through the pelvic inlet and not much happens, now, beyond the widening of the cervical canal, as the bag of waters is forced down by the squeezing of the uterus each time that it contracts. (See Fig. 23.) As the contractions grow stronger and more frequent you may have a desire to help matters by "bearing down," or straining, but this is very unwise for nothing that you can do will hasten the dilation of the cervix. The bearing down will tire you and then you will not be able to make as much helpful effort during the second stage as you would in a fresh and rested condition. For this reason, if your pains begin at night, don't get up, but stay in bed and try to get as much sleep as possible. If they begin during the day, keep up and about during most of the time, but lie down often enough and long enough to prevent your getting tired. But above all don't bear down during the first stage.

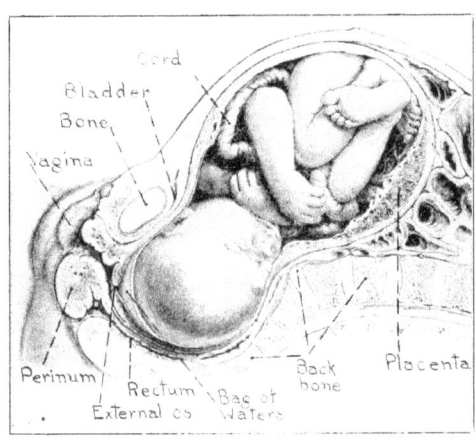

Fig. 23.—Drawing showing the baby's descent at the time of birth. The head is passing through the inlet and pressure by the bag of waters has started to dilate the cervix. (Drawn by Max Brödel. Used by permission of A. J. Nystrom and Co., Chicago.)

Take a warm soapsuds enema; a thorough, warm, sponge or shower bath, scrubbing the inner surface of the thighs and lower abdomen thoroughly, but do not bathe between the labia. Put on a freshly laundered nightgown, stockings, dressing-gown and slippers and braid your hair, preferably in two braids.

Drink all of the water you want and about every three or four hours take some form of liquid nourishment such as milk, cocoa, strained soup or broth, with toast or crackers. Such nourishment will help to keep you from getting tired and will do no harm, but it may not be altogether wise to take anything more solid without your doctor's permission. It is not uncommon for one to feel nauseated toward the end of the first stage and this tendency may be aggravated by taking solid food.

One thing to remember is the very great importance of your poise and favorable mental attitude. So much of proved value has been done, and still is being done, to safeguard you and your baby, that you have every reason to feel calm and secure, and it is of very practical importance that you cultivate this attitude. The woman who allows herself to become excited, nervous and apprehensive has much harder time than the one who asserts her self-mastery and preserves a tranquil state of mind. This is so definitely the case that for the sake of your own comfort I cannot urge you too strongly to remember it and to exclude disturbing or exciting influences as far as possible. One of the most troublesome of these is excitable but well-meaning and officious friends or relatives. Accordingly, if your nurse is not at hand try to have some one cool-headed woman with you and insist upon excluding those who would be upsetting or likely to offer advice and suggestions. In getting yourself ready, then, it is advisable to take a bath and an enema; put on clean clothing; not to stay in bed entirely throughout the first stage, but on the other hand to try to keep mind and body fresh and rested by lying down when you begin to feel tired, taking light nourishment regularly, not bearing down during pains and denying yourself to visitors who might be excitable.

This is all simple enough and you will not find it difficult to carry it out. And, happily, the preparations relating to the room are equally simple and uncomplicated.

Either you or the friend who is with you, may make the bed—you if you feel like it, she, if you are tired. The mattress is covered with the larger of the two pieces of rubber sheeting that you have in readiness and over this is placed the lower sheet, stretched very smooth and tight and tucked well under the mattress at head, foot and sides. If the sheet is not very large, it may be made secure by being pinned with safety-pins to the under side of the mattress. The smaller rubber is then placed across the middle third of the bed and over this a muslin sheet, folded once through the middle, tucked well under the sides of the mattress. Next, the upper sheet, a light blanket and a thin counterpane, all left open at the foot, and a pillow.

The packages of sterile dressings, douche pan, fountain syringe, pitchers and basins may be placed on the tables, and the washstand equipped for the doctor's hands with soap, sterile nail-brush, nail scissors and file. A large kettle or pail of water should be boiled, covered and put aside to cool and a large receptacle such as a wash-boiler, half or two thirds full of water put on to boil when the pains begin to come about every five minutes.

The baby's bathtub should be near at hand for sometimes babies do not breathe quite satisfactorily at first and are helped to do so by being held in a tub of warm water. There should be, also, a box, basket or crib, in readiness to receive the baby, furnished with a clean blanket and hot water bottle with a flannel cover.

These are the preparations which may be made during the first stage—that period when the cervix is being slowly but steadily dilated by the bag of waters as it is forced downward by the uterine contractions. You feel these as pains beginning in the back, and finally in the lower abdomen and thighs, gradually growing stronger and more frequent.

Second Stage. The first stage is ended, and the second stage begins, when the cervix is wide enough for the baby to pass through. From this time on you should stay in bed and if neither the doctor nor the nurse has arrived, your cool-headed friend must stand by and not leave you alone. The bag of waters usually, though not always, breaks at this time, and there is a rush of fluid. But the character of the pains changes even though the membranes do not rupture. They come about every two minutes, now, from the beginning of one pain to the one following, each pain lasting about a minute. They are stronger and more forcible and you begin to have an uncontrollable desire to strain or bear down.

If the doctor or nurse is with you, they will tell you how to use your pains to advantage, but if they are not there you would better avoid bearing down since you want to retard the baby's birth, if possible, until one or the other arrives. In such a case, you may delay matters by opening your mouth and breathing deeply during pains and by lying on your side.

We all know that in spite of the most careful planning, babies are sometimes born before the arrival of doctor or nurse and that the mother and her cool-headed friend, who is standing by, meet the emergency together. Fortunately, births occurring under such circumstances are not the ones that are likely to be associated with trouble for either mother or baby, so there is little or no cause for concern. Most doctors feel that the wisest course for the cool-headed friend to follow at such a time is to do nothing at all. So if the baby arrives in advance of the doctor, why, he is here, and that is about all there is to it! The moment you have been longing for, for nine long months, has come; your anxiety and waiting are all over, and with much less trouble than you expected.

Third Stage. After the baby is born, your pains will subside for a few moments and then the uterus will begin again to contract and gradually detach the placenta from its inner surface, forcing it out just as the baby was expelled.

In the meantime the baby is lying on the foot of the bed with the cord connecting him with the placenta which is still within your uterus. Under no circumstances should anyone pull on the cord to aid in the expulsion of the placenta. It will come away, naturally, in due time. When the placenta is finally expelled, the third and last stage of labor is over.

In case you and your cool-headed friend feel that something should be done, perhaps I would better assure you once more that when a baby is born so quickly and easily that he arrives before the doctor, you have cause for relief only—not anxiety. Practically the only unfavorable conditions which may arise are hemorrhage in your case and failure to breathe satisfactorily, on the part of the baby, and you and your cool-headed friend may as well understand how simply these possibilities may be met.

Although, as everyone knows, there is normally a certain amount of blood lost at the time of confinement, varying from one half to one pint, this is accepted as a matter of course. A serious hemorrhage very rarely occurs because of one of Nature's ingenious provisions. The tiny muscle fibers that make up the uterine wall run in every direction, criss-cross, up and down and around, forming a veritable tangle. After the placenta comes away, all of these little fibers contract, or grow shorter, and the result is that the muscles squeeze down upon the blood-vessels so tightly that they are closed and blood cannot escape.

Accordingly, as long as the uterine muscles are contracted there can be no hemorrhage. The fortunate thing about this is that you can find out if they are contracted, and if they are not, you, yourself can stimulate them to do so. If you will press your fingers down deep into your abdomen, near the navel, you will feel the uterus as a hard round mass, which is often likened to a baseball. If it continues to feel hard and round there cannot be any serious amount of bleeding, but if it becomes soft, the tiny muscle fibers are relaxing their grip on the vessels and bleeding may possibly occur. Quite naturally the thing to do, then, is to stimulate the muscles to contract and this is done by kneading the uterus through the abdominal wall. You will feel it grow hard under your hand and then you will know that everything is all right.

Your friend may want to bathe you and put on a pad but it would be better to leave this for the doctor or nurse for this reason: Childbed fever is the result of introducing infective material into the vagina. Remember that. If no germs gain entrance, there will be no childbed fever. When your baby came quickly and there was a rush of water, your vagina was well washed out. If you and your friend keep fingers and everything else away from the vaginal outlet and the area immediately surrounding it, it will remain clean and you need not worry about the possibility of infection.

Perhaps I have given more space to all of this than seems warrantable, but I want you to know just what is going on so that you will not be worried. And also, in order that you will not make trouble for yourself by trying to do something when all that you really need do is to lie still, as comfortably as possible, keep your hand on the uterus and knead it enough to keep it hard.

If your friend can slip out the wet sheet and put a dry one in its place, without your having to turn over, you will be just that much more comfortable, but the doctor will attend to everything else when he comes.

Next the baby. Presumably he is lying there on the foot of the bed, all safe and sound, trying to get used to the new order of things. He is probably making his presence known by crying lustily and though the day may come when that sound will not be altogether pleasant, it is nothing short of music to you now, for you have been waiting a long time to hear it. The baby has come from a very warm place and has suddenly undergone the most abrupt change in his entire mode of living that he will ever experience, so the transition should be made as easy for him as possible. There are two things which he must do immediately, that your body has been doing for him. He must breathe through his lungs and he must keep his body warm. If he has cried loudly, your faithful cool-headed friend may just wrap a little blanket about him, letting him lie as he is until the doctor comes, taking care that his face is not covered for he needs plenty of air. If the room is chilly she might place a flannel covered bag of warm water beside him outside the blanket.

If the baby has not really cried lustily, as we know that even the youngest baby can, he should be made to cry, as that is the way he gets his breathing apparatus to running as it should. Your friend may take one of the clean little gauze squares that you prepared, and wrapping it around her little finger reach well back into the baby's mouth and remove any mucus that may be lodged there and interfere with his breathing. She will do this more easily and thoroughly if she will pick the baby up by the feet, with one finger between his slippery little ankles so that her grip will be firm, and wipe out his mouth as he hangs head down.

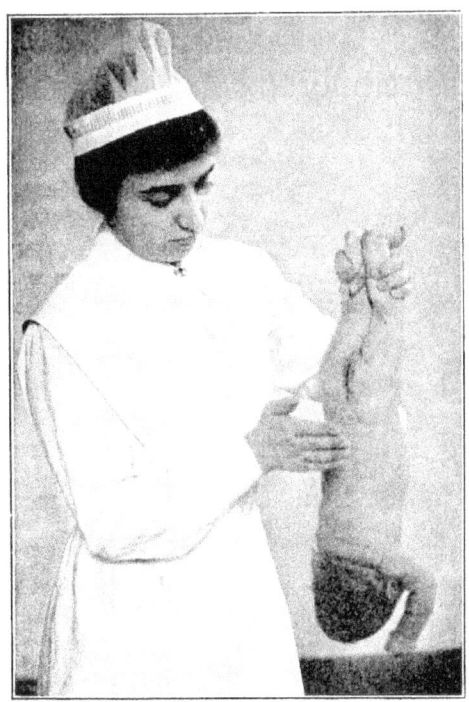

FIG. 24.—Helping the new baby to breathe by holding him head downward and sharply spanking him. Note that the nurse has one finger between the baby's ankles to prevent his slipping from her hand.

The main thing to remember is that the lining of that new little mouth is as delicate as a rose leaf and if it is wiped with other than the gentlest stroke the surface may be injured and give trouble later on. While he is hanging, head down, your friend may rub his back or stroke it with her free hand and in all probability you will then hear the baby use his lungs to your heart's content. But if he still does not cry well he may be sharply spanked two or three times as shown in Fig. 24. In this picture the cord has been cut and the baby is removed from the bed, but that is not necessary for it is very common to hold the baby up, wipe out his mouth, stroke his back or spank him, before the cord is cut.

You need not be at all disturbed if your baby needs these little forms of encouragement, at first, for remember that all of a sudden he is given some very complicated and taxing work to do and it is only reasonable that he should have all possible help as he undertakes it.

Remember, too, in looking forward to this event, that the probability that you or your friend will have to think of any of these things is very remote for the doctor and nurse are almost certain to be with you, and you will be able to give yourself over entirely to being very happy that at last your baby has come.

THE MIRACLE[1]

By

Elizabeth Newport Hepburn

The wind blows down the street,
   A shutter bangs somewhere,
While twilight falls as softly as
   A woman's flowing hair.

Within a quiet room,
   Adventurers at rest,
A mother holds her new-born son,
   Safe, now, upon her breast!

For out of Night and Pain,
   The womb of mystery,
Is sprung this miracle of Life
   That she can touch and see.

No seer's prophetic dream,
   No star in all the skies
Burns with a luster half so bright
   As happy mother eyes.

No questor for the Grail,
   No searcher for the Truth,
Counts more than those who bear and rear
   And love and nurture Youth!

Within her curving arm,
   All safe and warm he lies,
The heir of all that Man has won
   Down countless centuries!

  1. Written expressly for "Obstetrical Nursing" by Carolyn Conant Van Blarcom.

CHAPTER VIII
THE BABY'S MOTHER

For the first week or two after the baby comes, you will be in bed, of course; your doctor will come in often and you will doubtless be cared for by a nurse devoted exclusively to you, or by a visiting nurse aided by members of your family. You will find that it is money well spent to keep the nurse, or someone else, to care for and help you, for six or eight weeks after the baby's birth, or longer if possible.

Adequate care after childbirth accomplishes two important ends. It practically always averts such immediate complications as hemorrhage and infection and it prevents more or less chronic invalidism. Infection is prevented by the scrupulously clean care which is given to your breasts and perineum, while hemorrhage is avoided by keeping you quiet and closely watching the condition of the uterus. Later invalidism is prevented by the many precautions which enter into your general care. These relate to your position in bed, diet, fresh air, rest, exercise, bathing, attention to your bowels; observance of symptoms and conserving all of your forces while increasing your strength.

All of these details are important, for during the five or six weeks after confinement certain changes take place in your body which return it very nearly to its pre-pregnant state, and lack of watchful care while these changes are in progress may retard them and result in your being more or less permanently wretched.

Make every effort, therefore, to secure the care that you need during this transitional period of five or six weeks called the *puerperium*.

You will doubtless feel a little tired and nervous at first, for you have been through something of an ordeal, but when one considers the great things that your body has accomplished, your recovery and return to a normal condition will be surprisingly rapid. During the first few days you are likely to have little or no appetite but be very thirsty; be constipated; perspire freely and have an increased amount of urine, which you may have difficulty in passing; but these conditions are only temporary.

In the beginning you will probably be nursed just about as anyone would be after a slight operation, with the addition of special attention to your breasts and perineum to prevent infection, and the toning up of abdominal muscles. In order to prevent bleeding and hasten your recovery you will be kept very quiet for a day or two, perhaps flat on your back; you may not be allowed to have any visitors and your diet, at first consisting of liquids, will finally be made up of light, easily digestible but nourishing food.

About the sixth or eighth day you will probably begin to sit up in bed and about the ninth or tenth day you may be allowed to sit up in a chair for a little while. Some young mothers are able to sit up for an hour the first time, without fatigue, while others can sit up for only a few moments, morning and afternoon, on the first day, gradually lengthening the period each time that they get up. You will probably be able to sit up an hour or so longer on each successive day and walk a few steps on the third or fourth day after getting up.

These first few days of being up and trying to walk are often tiring, and a little discouraging in consequence, but of course you will gain steadily, even though it be slowly, do a little more each day and gradually feel more and more like your old self.

The mother who has stitches, because of the perineum having been torn at the time of the baby's birth, does not usually sit up in bed until the ninth or tenth day, when the stitches are removed, sitting up in a chair for an hour, two or three days later. In connection with tears it may be well for you to know that in spite of the most skillful and careful efforts to prevent them, tears of some degree usually occur when the first baby is born and in about half of the confinements that follow.

But as most tears are very slight and are immediately repaired they have little or no effect upon one's comfort or general health.

It is ordinarily considered a safe precaution to avoid going up and down stairs until the baby is about four weeks old and not wholly to resume normal activities within six or eight weeks after his birth. A pinkish or red discharge or backache, after the mother gets up are regarded as indications that she is not quite ready to do much standing or walking and that she still needs a good deal of rest.

The whole question of the time for sitting up, of getting up and of walking about varies so with different individuals, as you see, that it is not possible to describe a definite routine, for some women recover slowly and would be injured by getting up and about at a period which would be entirely safe and normal for the majority. The doctor has to decide what is best in each case.

While you are being actually nursed as a bed patient, especial attention is given to the bathing of the perineum, as has been stated; the care of the breasts and restoring tone to your abdominal muscles, so we may well have a word of explanation about each of these details.

The Perineum. The nurse will bathe the area between your thighs very carefully, at regular intervals, using pledgets soaked in some kind of antiseptic solution, and put on a fresh one of the sterile pads that you made and sterilized some weeks back. This attention is partly to promote your comfort and partly to remove any infective material that may be present, thus preventing fever. After the care that you have had up to this time, it will scarcely be possible for you to have childbed fever if all infective material is kept away from the vaginal outlet. I speak of this in order that you may realize how important it is for you to avoid touching these parts with your fingers, upon which there are almost certain to be germs. There is little doubt that women sometimes seriously infect themselves after the doctor and nurse have taken the most scrupulous care to protect them from this very complication.

Your **breasts** will be given painstaking care in order that the baby may nurse satisfactorily and to prevent both sore nipples and breast abscesses. If you cared for your breasts during the latter part of pregnancy as was advised in Chapter V and will continue to observe ordinary precautions while the baby is nursing, it is not at all likely that you will have any trouble with your breasts.

The main features of the care of your breasts, now, are keeping the nipples clean and supporting the breasts themselves if they grow heavy enough to be uncomfortable. This latter condition is not uncommon about the third or fourth day after the baby is born, when the colostrum is replaced by what one might call almost a rush of milk. The breasts may then become hard, swollen and uncomfortable and sometimes a sensitive lump or "cake" may be felt. The usual course, nowadays is simply to support those swollen breasts and to apply ice bags or hot compresses to the painful areas.

There are innumerable bandages and methods for supporting heavy breasts, any one of which is satisfactory so long as it meets the two chief requirements: to lift the breasts, suspending their weight from the shoulders, and, while fitting snugly below, to avoid making pressure at any point, particularly over the nipples. One may take a towel for example, or a straight strip of muslin, fasten it around the chest, pin in darts below the breasts with safety-pins, and provide support by means of shoulder straps, attached with safety-pins to the front and back of the binder. Fig. 25 shows such a binder being used to hold ice bags in place, for which also it is satisfactory and very easily devised.

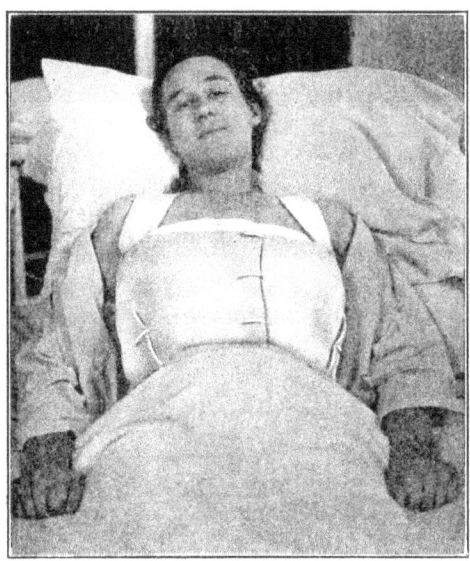

FIG. 25.—Straight binder for supporting heavy breasts, or holding ice caps in place on breasts that are painful. Darts are pinned in below the breasts and the binder is held up by shoulder straps, pinned on front and back.

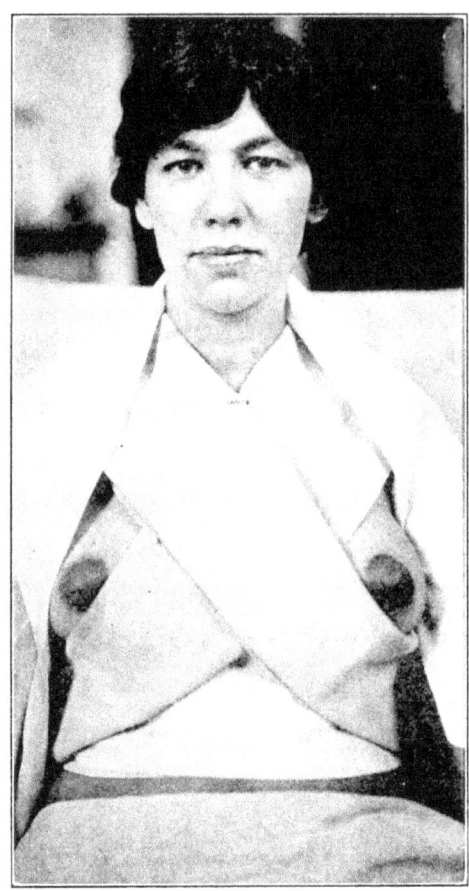

Fig. 26.—Supporting heavy breasts by means of three folded towels; one fastened about the waist, one over each shoulder, crossing front and back.

Three folded towels or folded bands of muslin will provide a comfortable support if applied in the sling-like manner indicated in Fig. 26; the Indian binder shown in Fig. 27, made of cheesecloth or any soft material is cool, light and very comfortable, and in addition to these improvised binders there are several entirely satisfactory brassières, opening down the front, to be bought in the shops. Happily the discomfort from swollen breasts lasts only a day or two, for in some mysterious way Nature makes an adjustment between the amount of milk produced by the mother and that withdrawn by the baby. So as he comes to nurse regularly and satisfactorily, the excessive supply of milk disappears, and with it the discomfort.

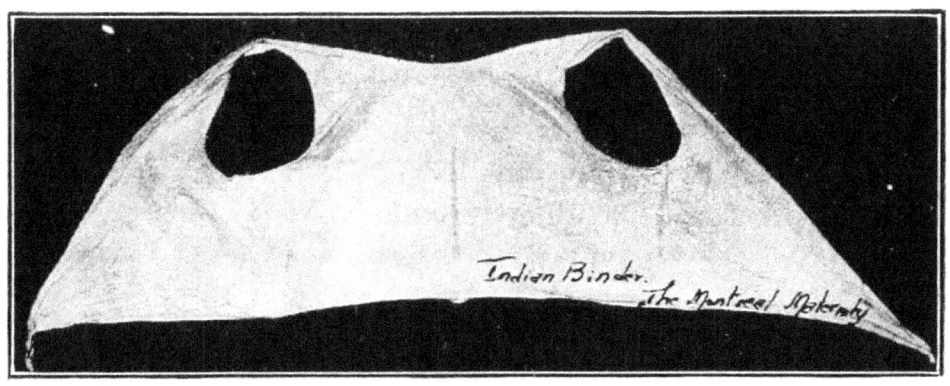

Fig. 27.—Indian binder for supporting heavy breasts, used at The Montreal Maternity Hospital. The tapering ends tie in a knot in front.

The care of the nipples practically resolves itself into keeping them clean in order to avoid infection. Notice that I say *keeping* them clean, for merely bathing them, no matter how regularly, is not enough. The nurse will probably bathe your nipples with boracic acid solution and sterile cotton pledgets before and after each time that the baby nurses, and keep them covered, during the intervals, with sterile gauze or cotton.

Here again you may undo all of the nurse's careful precautions against infection, which might cause an abscess, if you touch your nipples with your fingers or anything else that is not sterile, except the baby's mouth. The gauze squares or sponges or the cotton pledgets that you sterilized will serve excellently to protect your nipples between nursings. These may be held in place by a binder or by tapes tied through the ends of narrow strips of adhesive plaster, four being applied to each breast as shown in Fig. 28. Strips of adhesive plaster about five inches long are folded back at one end so that two adhesive surfaces stick together for about an inch. Through a hole cut in this folded end a narrow tape or bobbin is tied, and the strips are applied to the breast, beginning at the margin of the darkened area and extending outward. The free ends of the tapes are tied over pads of gauze or cotton between nursings, and untied to expose the nipple at nursing time.

Lead shields are sometimes used to protect the nipples, being held in place by means of a binder. These shields should be scoured and boiled daily.

Method of Nursing. One important reason for all of this scrupulous care is that it favors the baby's nursing satisfactorily and without interruption, so now you will want to know about the actual details of nursing him.

The baby is usually put to the breast for the first time, between eight and twelve hours after he is born. This gives the mother an opportunity to rest, and the baby too profits by being quiet and undisturbed during this interval. His need for food is not great as yet, nor is there much if any nourishment available for him. There is no hard and fast rule for the mother's position in bed, while nursing her baby, beyond the fact that both she and the infant should be in a relation that makes the nursing easy. One very natural and satisfactory method is for her to turn slightly to one side, and hold the baby in the curve of her arm so that he may easily grasp the nipple on that side. If you take this position you should hold your breast from the baby's face with your free hand by placing the thumb above and the fingers below the nipple, thus leaving his nose uncovered to permit free breathing, as shown in Fig. 29. You and the baby should lie in such positions that both will be comfortable and relaxed and the baby will be able to take into his mouth, not only the nipple but much of the dark circle as well, so as to compress the base of the nipple with his jaws and extract the milk by suction.

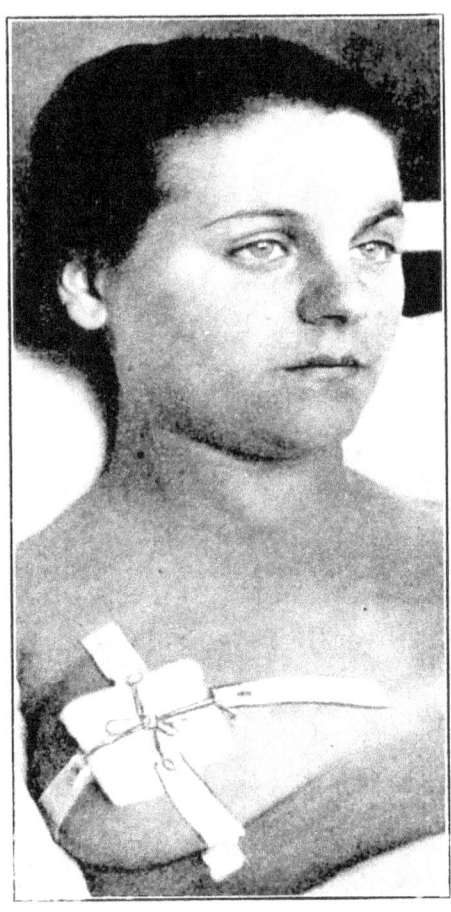

FIG. 28.—Sterile gauze held in place over nipples by means of tapes and adhesive strips.

The comfort of this position is sometimes increased by laying the baby on a small pillow placed close to the mother's side, thus raising his body to the level of his head as it rests upon her arm.

You and the nurse may have to resort to a number of expedients in persuading the baby to begin to nurse, for he does not always take the breast eagerly at first. He must be kept awake, first and foremost, and sometimes suckling will be encouraged by patting or stroking his cheek or chin or lightly spanking his buttocks. If his head is drawn away from the breast a little, as he holds the nipple in his mouth, he will sometimes take a firmer hold and begin to nurse. Moistening the nipple by expressing a few drops of colostrum or with sweetened water may whet the baby's appetite and thus prompt him to nurse.

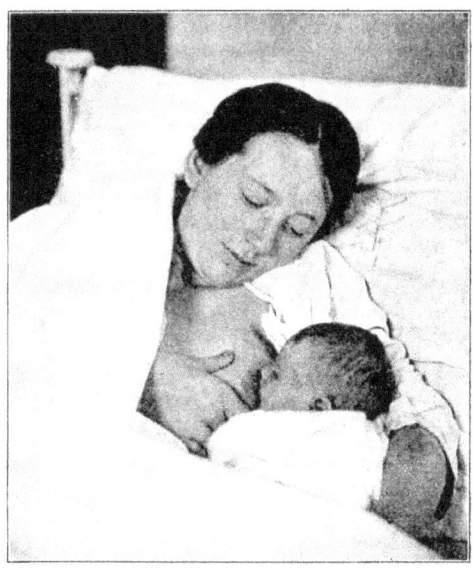

FIG. 29.—A comfortable position for mother and baby, while nursing in bed.

You must be prepared to find the early attempts to nurse your baby far from satisfactory, but if you persevere in making attempts regularly, you will almost certainly succeed.

During the first two or three days the baby obtains only colostrum while nursing, but the regular suckling is extremely important, not alone for the sake of getting him into the habit of nursing but because his suckling is the best and surest means of stimulating your breasts to produce milk. And, as we shall see in a moment, the irritation of the nipples in this manner so definitely promotes desirable changes in the uterus that these go on more rapidly in women who nurse their babies than in those who do not.

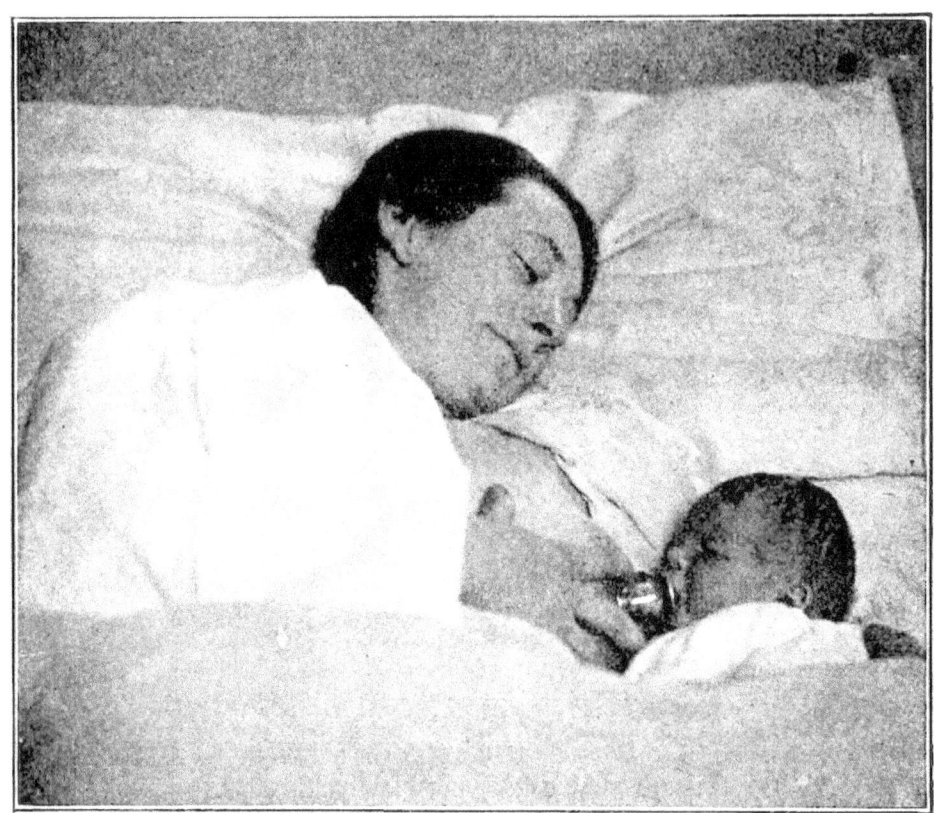

Fig. 30.—Protecting cracked or sore nipples by having the baby nurse through a shield.

If your nipples are not sufficiently prominent for the baby to grasp them, or if they become sore, you may have to use a shield for a while as shown in Figs. 30 and 31, but the shield should be discarded as soon as possible for it is the baby's suckling that produces the desired effects. If a shield is used, it should be washed and boiled after each nursing and kept in a sterile jar or solution of boracic acid, between times.

The length of the nursing periods, and the intervals between them, are decided upon by the doctor according to the needs and condition of each baby: his weight, vigor, the rapidity with which he nurses, the character of his stools and his general condition. The length of the nursing periods themselves, is usually from ten to twenty minutes, the intervals between them being measured from the beginning of one feeding to the beginning of the next, and are fairly uniform for babies of the same age and weight.

The average baby nurses about every six hours during the first two days, or four times in twenty-four hours. After this, according to one schedule, he will nurse every three hours during the day for about three months and at 10 p.m. and 2 a.m., or seven times in twenty-four hours. From the third to the sixth month he nurses every three hours during the day and at ten o'clock at night, or six times in twenty-four hours, and from that time until he is weaned he nurses at four-hour intervals during the day and at ten o'clock at night, or five times daily. Such a feeding schedule may be arranged in a table as follows:

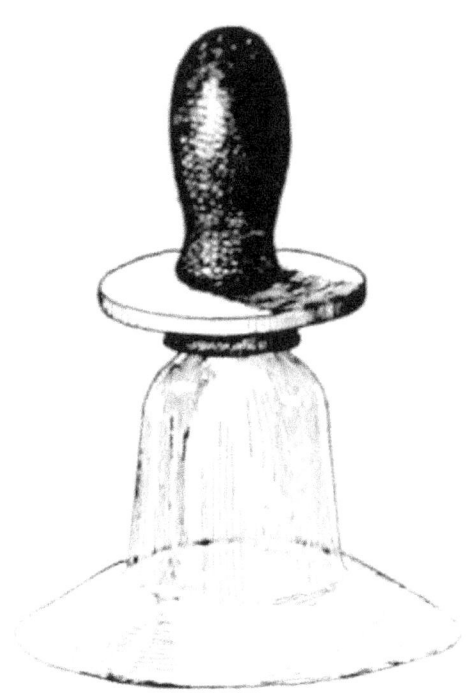

Fig. 31.—Nipple shield used in Fig. 30.

	Day					Night	
First and second days	6	12	6			12	
First three months	6	9	12	3	6	10	2 a.m.
Third to sixth month	6	9	12	3	6	10	
After the sixth month	6	10	2	6		10	

It is becoming more and more common to omit night feedings after ten o'clock with the average baby who is in good condition even during the first three months. When this practice is adopted the baby seems not only to do as well as he normally should, but to profit by the long digestive rest during the night. Certainly the mother is benefited by the unbroken sleep thus made possible.

As a rule the baby nurses from one side, only, at each nursing, emptying the breasts alternately, but if there is not enough milk in one breast for a complete feeding both breasts may be used at one nursing. Neither you nor the baby should go to sleep while he is at the breast, but he should pause every four or five minutes to keep him from feeding too rapidly.

After you sit up you will find it a good plan to occupy a low, comfortable chair while nursing the baby. Lean slightly forward and raise the knee upon which the baby rests by placing your foot on a stool; support his head in the curve of your arm and hold your breast from his face though slightly above it, just as you did while nursing him in bed. Nurse him in a quiet room where you will not be disturbed and where neither your breasts nor the baby will be exposed to drafts or the possibility of being chilled.

Some mothers like to lie down while nursing the baby, for in addition to finding the position comfortable they are glad to have these regular, though short periods of rest.

Abdominal Binders and Bed-Exercises. Most women are interested in this question as it concerns the restoration or preservation of the "figure."

The application of a snug binder for the first day or two after the baby comes, is a fairly common practice, for many women are very uncomfortable as a result of the sudden release of tension on their abdominal walls, a discomfort which a binder relieves. And during the first few days after the mother gets up and walks about she is sometimes given great comfort by a binder that is put on and snugly adjusted about her hips and the lower part of her abdomen, as she lies on her back.

In addition to this, some doctors like to have the young mother wear a snug binder throughout her entire stay in bed, while others instruct their patients to take bed exercises. If the binder is your portion, you have nothing to do but wear it, for some one else must put it on you. But if bed exercises are in order, the following descriptions and pictures of the exercises taken by young mothers at the Long Island College Hospital may be helpful.

The day upon which the exercises are started, the rate at which they are increased and the length of time during which they are continued, are, of course, entirely regulated by the doctor according to the strength and needs of each patient, for they are never continued to the point of fatigue. Quite evidently, then, there can be no definite directions for these exercises; one can give only a description of the positions and movements that are frequently used and the order in which they are adopted.

The average mother who is recovering normally begins the chin-to-chest exercise from twelve to twenty-four hours after the baby's birth. She lies flat on her back and raises her head until the chin rests upon her chest. (See Fig. [32](#).) By resting her hand upon the abdomen she feels for herself that the abdominal muscles contract as she lifts her head and accordingly realizes that she is actually exercising them. The movement is usually repeated twenty-five times, morning and evening, every day and continued as long as the patient is in bed.

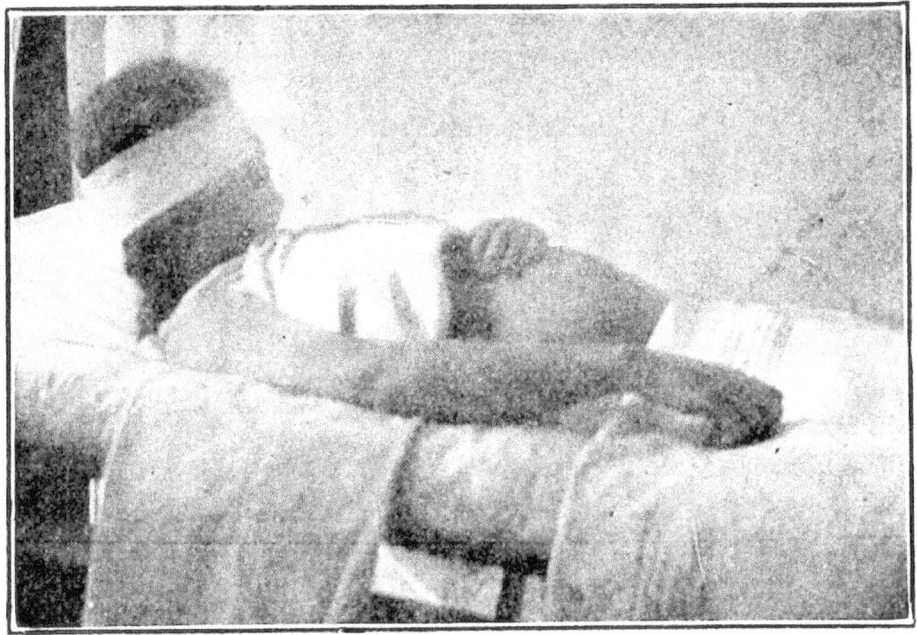

Fig. 32.

Figs. 32 to 38 inclusive are bed exercises the young mother. For description see text. (From photographs taken at the Long Island College Hospital.)

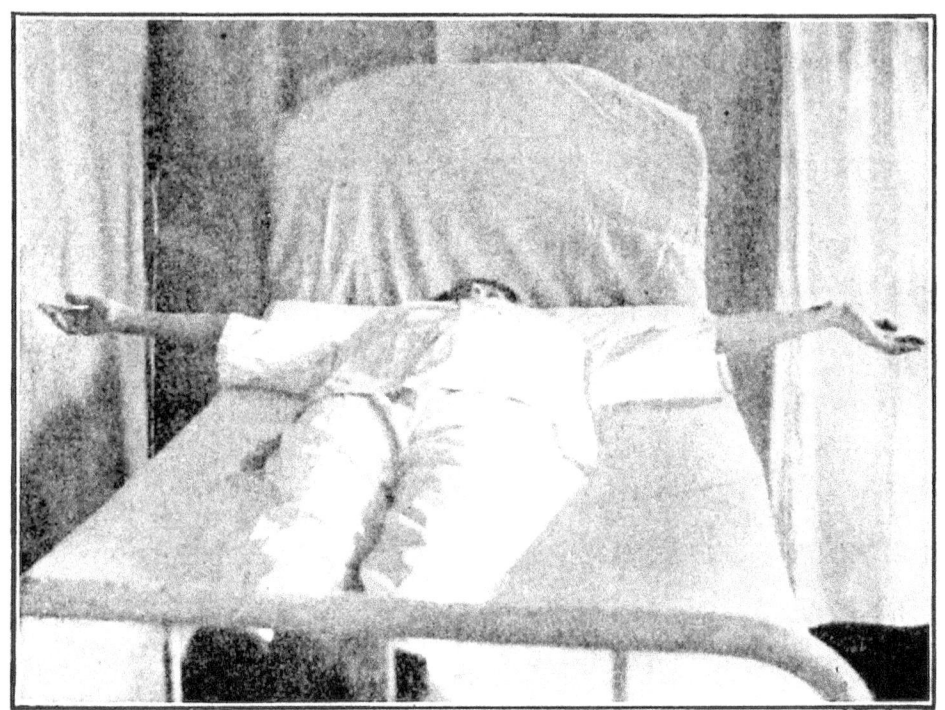

Fig. 33.

The familiar deep-breathing exercise comes next and is ordinarily started on the third or fourth day. The mother lies flat, with her arms at her sides, then extends them straight out from the shoulders (Fig. 33), raises them above her head, as in Fig. 34, and returns them to their original position. She repeats this exercise ten times morning and evening as long as she is in bed.

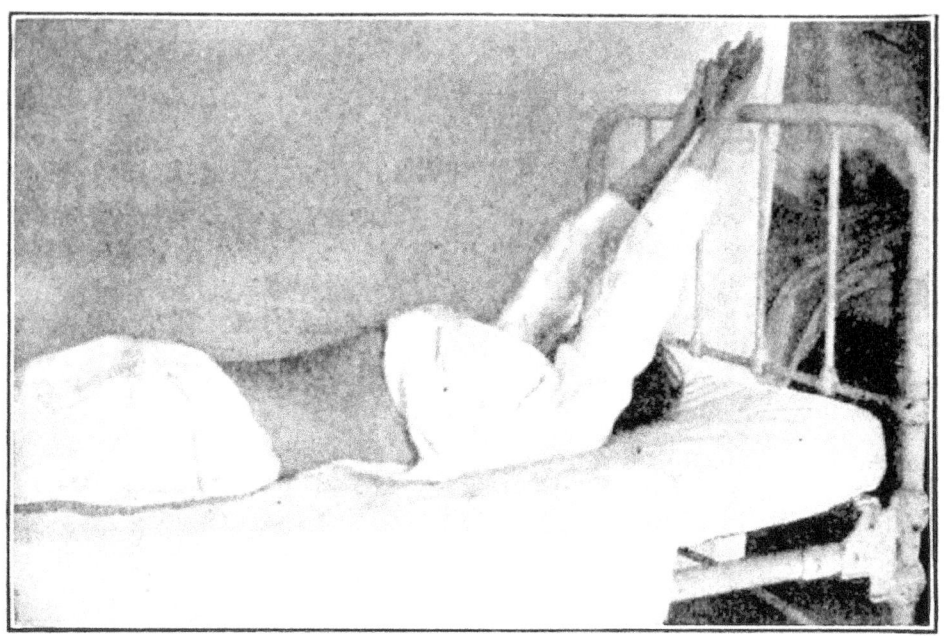

FIG. 34.

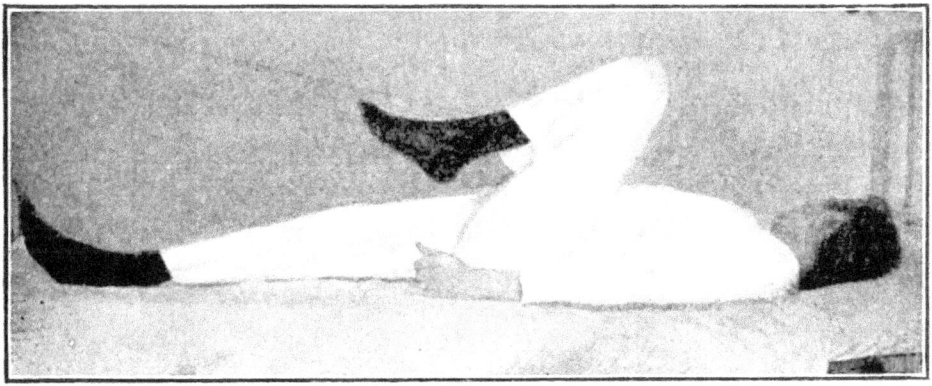

FIG. 35.

The one-leg flexion exercises are not taken by mothers who have stitches, but in other cases they are usually started about the fifth day. One thigh is flexed sharply on the abdomen and the foot brought down to the buttocks as in Fig. 35. The leg is then straightened out and lowered to the bed. This is repeated ten times, with each leg, morning and evening, for two or three days.

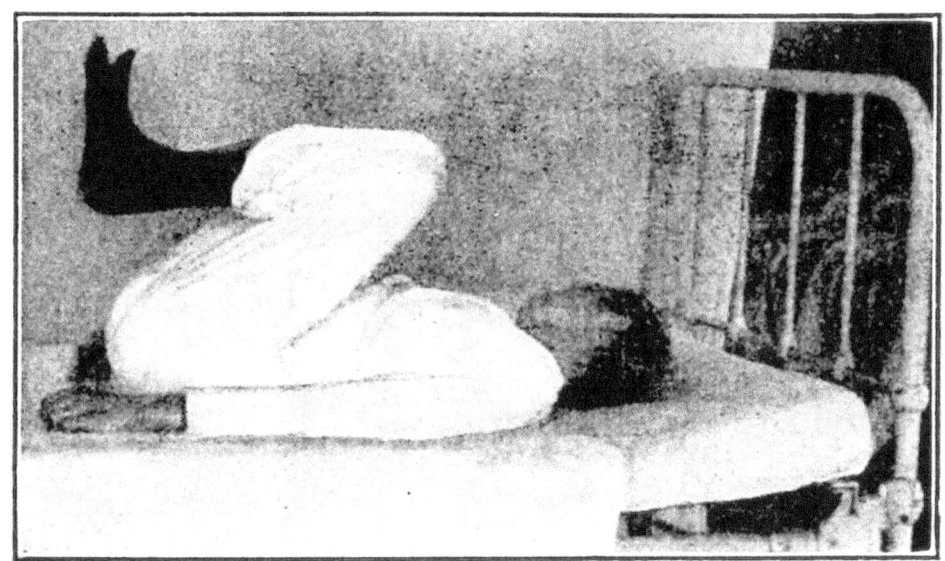

Fig. 36.

The next exercise sometimes replaces the one-leg-flexion and sometimes it is taken up in addition to it, being started after the former has been done for a day or two, according to the strength of the mother. Both thighs are brought up on the abdomen in this one, as in Fig. 36, but when the legs are straightened the feet are lowered not quite to the bed, as in Fig. 37, before being raised again. This is repeated ten times morning and evening.

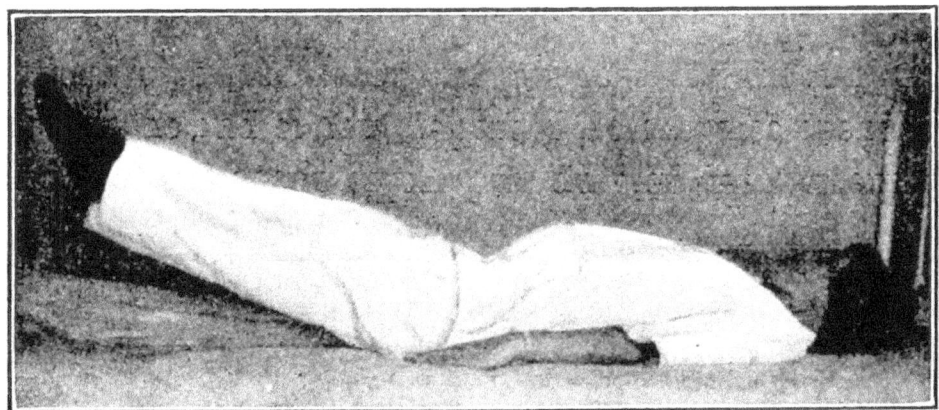

Fig. 37.

Then comes the exercise for which the leg-flexions prepare the mother and which are sometimes discontinued when this one is adopted. It is started, as a rule, about the seventh day, or two or three days before the mother gets up. Both legs are slowly raised to a position at right angles to the body, as in Fig. 38, and slowly lowered but not far enough for the heels to touch the bed (see Fig. 37), and the movement repeated. As this exercise requires a good deal of effort it is taken up very gradually, somewhat as follows: The legs are raised once in the morning and twice in the evening of the first day; second day, three times in the morning and four times in the evening; third day, five times in the morning and six times in the evening and so on, if the mother is not fatigued, until the exercise is repeated ten times or more each morning and evening for several months.

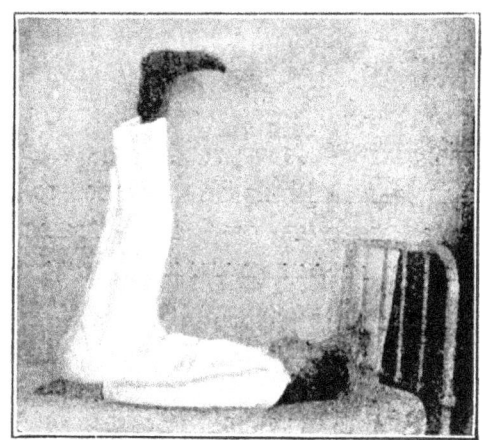

Fig. 38.

The **knee chest position** shown in Fig. 39 is intended to prevent a misplacement of the uterus, from which so many women suffer after childbirth. It is usually started about the seventh day and the patient begins by being assisted to that position and keeping it for a moment or two, gradually lengthening the time to about five minutes each morning and evening; this is often continued for two months or more.

Walking on all fours is violent exercise and is taken up very gradually. Some women are able to attempt it on the first day out of bed, if they have been taking the other exercises regularly, but as a rule it is not started until the second, third or fourth day after getting up. The clothes are free from all constrictions, pajamas being very satisfactory; the knees are held stiff and straight with the feet widely separated, to allow a rush of air into the vagina, and the entire palmar surface of the hands rests flat on the floor. (See Fig. 40.) The patient starts by taking only a few steps each morning and evening, gradually lengthening the walk to five minutes twice daily and continuing it for about two months. It is believed that as the young mother walks in this position the uterus and rectum rub against each other, producing something the same result as would be obtained if it were possible to massage them, the effect of this being to promote involution, which will be explained later, and lessen the tendency toward constipation and uterine misplacement.

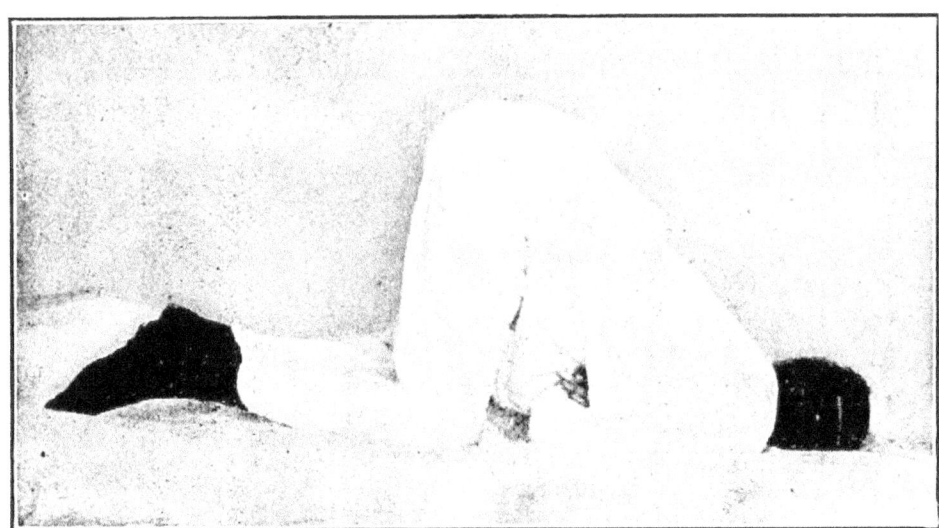

Fig. 39.—Knee chest position.

The general purpose of these exercises, as a whole, then, is to strengthen the abdominal muscles, thus helping to prevent a large, pendulous abdomen; to increase the convalescing mother's general strength and tone just as exercise benefits the average person; to promote involution (See page 134); to prevent misplacement of the uterus and in a measure to relieve constipation. In order that the exercises may accomplish these much-to-be-desired ends, the doctors who advise them feel that it is important for them to be taken with moderation and judgment; started slowly; increased gradually and constantly adjusted to the strength of the individual mother.

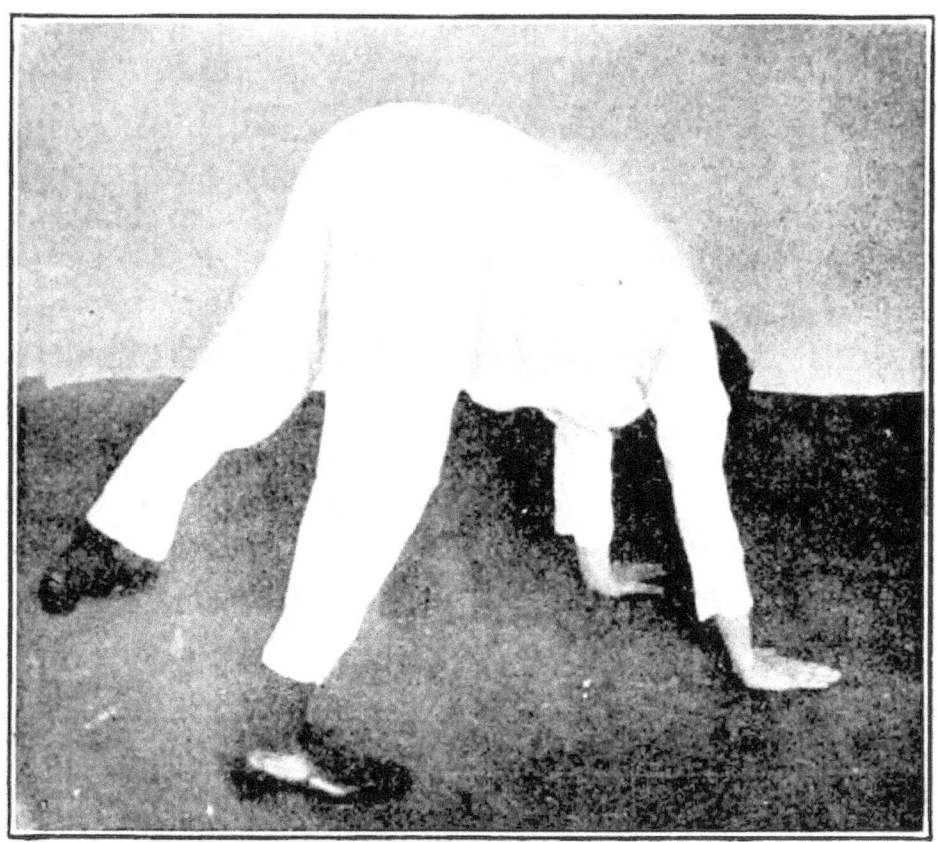

Fig. 40.—Walking on all fours.

Otherwise they may do more harm than good.

Concerning the changes that take place in your body during the puerperium, the ones that will interest you particularly are: (1) the shrinkage in the size of your uterus and its gradual descent into the pelvis where it was before the baby began his life within it; (2) the production of milk by your breasts; (3) a loss of body weight.

The Uterus. Immediately after delivery the uterus weighs about 2 pounds; is from 7 to 8 inches high; about 5 inches across and 4 inches thick. The top of the uterus, or fundus, may be felt just below the navel and the inner surface where the placenta was attached, is raw and bleeding. At the end of six or eight weeks the organ has descended into the pelvic cavity and resumed approximately its original position and size and its former weight of 2 ounces. This return of the uterus to practically its pre-pregnant state is called *involution* and in the interest of your immediate recovery and future health it is important that this shall progress normally.

There is evidently a close relation between the functions of the breasts and of the uterus and accordingly involution is likely to progress more satisfactorily in women who nurse their babies than in those who do not. The so-called "after-pains," also, are affected by nursing, being more severe, as a rule, when the baby is at the breast than at other times. These pains are caused by alternate contractions and relaxations of the uterine muscles and are more common in women who have had other children than after the first baby. These pains usually subside after the first twenty-four hours, though they may persist for three or four days.

In connection with the changes that take place in the uterus, the discharge called *lochia* should be mentioned. This is quite profuse and bloody at first but if the uterus involutes normally the discharge gradually decreases in amount and fades in color, until by the end of the puerperium it has entirely disappeared.

The Production of Milk. During the first two or three days after the baby is born, the breasts secrete a small amount of yellowish fluid called *colostrum*, which differs somewhat from the milk that comes later. About the third day the meager amount of colostrum is replaced by milk and as this increases rapidly in amount, the breasts usually become tense and swollen and sometimes painful; but this discomfort generally subsides in a day or two.

The production of milk is definitely stimulated by the baby's suckling and will not continue for more than a few days without this stimulation, a fact to be remembered if, for any reason, it is desirable to dry up the breasts. The end earnestly to be desired is for the breasts to produce a quantity and quality of milk which will adequately nourish the baby during the first eight or ten months of his life, and with proper care and effort this ideal can nearly always be realized. But if the mother becomes pregnant while nursing her baby—and this sometimes occurs as early as a few weeks after childbirth—the quality of her milk is likely to suffer.

The return of menstruation, however, does not necessarily affect the milk unfavorably, as is so generally believed. It is true that in the ideal course of events, the mother does not menstruate while nursing her baby, that is, for eight or ten months, but it is probable that about one-third of all nursing mothers begin to menstruate about two months after confinement and half of those who do not nurse their babies begin to menstruate in six weeks. A nursing mother may menstruate once and then not again for several months or a year; or she may menstruate regularly and still nurse her baby satisfactorily.

Menstruation is more likely to return early after the birth of the first baby than after those born subsequently. Mothers sometimes wonder whether this early discharge is menstrual or lochial, and though they, themselves, cannot possibly distinguish between them, a physician can easily decide by examination, and in the interest of the mother's future health it is important that this uncertainty be cleared up.

The loss of weight is one of the striking changes which take place during the puerperium, varying in different women from a total loss of from twelve to fifteen pounds. Fat women lose more than thin women and those who nurse their babies lose more than those who do not. This loss may be somewhat controlled, however, by suitable diet and under most conditions the mother returns to not less than her pre-pregnant weight by the end of the sixth or eighth week. You will recall that there was a general gain in weight, over the entire body, during pregnancy, in addition to the increased weight of the uterus.

If all goes well, your doctor may not call to see you regularly after the first couple of weeks, but he will probably want to make a thorough examination, sometime about five or six weeks after the baby's birth. As this examination is a very influential factor in securing your future health you should be sure to have it made. A slight abnormality, if detected at this time, may usually be corrected with little difficulty, but if allowed to persist may result in chronic invalidism, or necessitate an operation. In case the uterus is not properly involuted, for example, or the perineum is found to be flabby, a little more rest in bed is indicated; while a uterine misplacement, which seems to occur in about a third of all cases, usually may be corrected by the adjustment of a pessary. Quite evidently, then, it rests with the young mother to coöperate with the doctor in guarding against future ill health, or even operations, by having this final examination made and following whatever course he prescribes, as a result of his inspection.

Most of the discussion in this chapter relates to the care that is given to you by others, in preparing you to take up life anew, perhaps unaided, and assume the care of your baby. As we shall see in the next chapter, the care of your baby, for the next few months, is closely associated with the care which you take of yourself and the regulation of your daily life.

CHAPTER IX
THE MOTHER'S CARE OF HERSELF—FOR THE BABY'S SAKE

Now that you actually have your baby in your arms, soft and warm and lovely, you find yourself looking into those wide, wondering eyes of his and wanting nothing so much as to give him your protection.

If he could talk, as he looks back at you, I fancy your baby would tell you how much your care of him, during the months before he was born, has meant, and then he would beg you to stand by, very closely, for a few months more, until he is a little more used to being a separate person living outside your body.

"You have given me a wonderful start," he seems to tell you, "and now I want to go on and develop the best possible mind and body. I shall be able to do this if you will help me, for what you can give me now is of more importance than what all the rest of the people in the world can give. You can give me through your milk exactly the materials that Nature intends me to use to develop and build this partly finished body of mine, and to protect it from disease. Just tide me over this most difficult period of my life, and I'll be a credit to us both, not only as a baby but as a growing child and later as a robust man or woman, helping to do my share of the world's work. I'll have fine straight limbs to bear me on my way, a good brain to help me take a creditable place among people who count, and steady nerves I'll have, that will always be dependable. I'll put into reality the dreams that you and I are dreaming, and when I do, I'll look back to these early weeks and months and realize that I could not have done it but for you."

And so you look into the eyes of this baby of yours and pledge yourself to stand by and do for him all that lies in your power, realizing already that the keeping of that pledge is going to bring you, along with its demands, an endless and satisfying happiness; a consciousness that you are doing something indispensable to your baby's welfare that no one else in the world can do.

You know, now, that your baby's greatest single need for the next few months is satisfactory nursing at your breast, but you will be able to give him this only if your diet and general mode of living are favorable to the production of good milk.

Quite evidently, then, your big service to your baby, for a while, is largely a matter of caring for yourself.

It seldom happens that the mother who has had good prenatal care, followed by good care during and after labor, is unable to nurse her baby if she orders her own life in the way that is known to be necessary to promote and maintain the production of breast milk. The first essential is her real desire to nurse her baby, next, her appreciation of the continuous care of herself that is necessary to this end, and third her whole-hearted willingness to take such care, for her baby's sake.

It is safe to say that if the doctor and the nurse and the baby's mother all want him to nurse at the breast, and all do everything in their power to make this possible, they will almost invariably succeed. This assertion can scarcely be made too positively and we should never lose sight of the fact that if the baby is not breast-fed he is being defrauded, and in the vast majority of cases, because of insufficient effort on the part of those who are caring for him.

Practically the only conditions which doctors in general now recognize as sufficient reason for the mother's not nursing her baby are retracted nipples, tuberculosis, convulsions, severe heart or kidney trouble, certain acute infectious diseases such as typhoid fever, and the state of pregnancy.

When none of these conditions exist, a favorable frame of mind and a state of good nutrition are the two indispensable factors in establishing breast feeding and maintaining the production of a satisfactory quantity and quality of breast milk. These factors in turn are both affected by the mother's general mode of living.

Women with happy, cheerful dispositions usually nurse their babies satisfactorily, while those who worry and fret are likely to have an insufficient supply of milk or milk of a poor quality. In addition to this sustained influence exerted by the nursing mother's state of mind it is well to remember that the quality of milk that has been entirely satisfactory may be seriously injured, for the time being, by a fit of temper, fright, grief, anxiety or any marked emotional disturbance. Actual poisons seem to be created as a result of these emotions and they may affect the baby so unfavorably as to make it necessary to give him artificial food, temporarily, and empty the breasts by pumping or stripping before he begins to nurse again.

I realize that it is not easy entirely to reorganize your life and assume new and exacting duties, while recovering from an experience resembling an illness in some of its effects, and still remain calm, undiscouraged and perpetually cheerful. But each tiny victory that you accomplish in your attempt to achieve this end will bring such satisfaction that you will not count the cost. And the incomparable, always deepening happiness of watching your very own baby grow lovelier and sturdier, day by day, because of the things that you, and no one else, are doing, will make you deny, even to yourself, that anything you do is hard. Particularly will this be true if you repeatedly remind yourself that the satisfactorily breast-fed baby is much more likely to live through the difficult first year than is the bottle-fed baby, and also is much less susceptible to disease and infection.

We shall consider, for a moment, the more important details of the routine care that you should give yourself, for the baby's sake, and then we shall be ready for the pleasantest task of all—the actual care of the baby himself.

In general you should try to live just a normal, tranquil, unhurried kind of life that is unfailingly regular in its daily routine.

Diet. As was the case during pregnancy, the question of your diet is an important one. Throughout the entire nursing period your food should be such that it will nourish you and also aid in producing milk of a character that will meet the baby's needs, the needs of a growing, developing body. The best producer of such milk is a diet consisting largely of milk, eggs, "leafy" vegetables and fresh fruit, all taken with an appetite made keen by constant fresh air. Bear this in mind and it will keep you from putting your faith in so-called milk-producing foods and nostrums.

Your meals may well be made up from the groups of foods that are suitable for the expectant mother, as given in Chapter V. At this time, as during pregnancy, you should avoid all food that may produce any form of indigestion, but for the baby's sake now, as well as your own. While it is not generally believed by doctors of to-day, that there are many, if any, articles of diet which may in themselves injure the mother's milk, it is generally accepted that if her digestion is upset this may be, and usually is, bad for her milk and therefore bad for the baby.

Certain drugs are excreted through the milk and may affect the baby just as they would if administered to him directly, as for example alcohol and opium, from which morphine, heroin, codein, laudanum and paregoric are derived.

Although the old belief no longer holds sway, that certain substances from such highly flavored vegetables as onions, cabbages, turnips and garlic were excreted through the milk and upset the baby, it is definitely known that certain substances in certain foods are excreted through the milk to the baby's great advantage. It is necessary to the baby's well-being, therefore, that the nursing mother's diet shall include, regularly, those articles of food which contain these substances. These foods are milk, egg-yolk, glandular organs such as sweetbreads, kidneys and liver; the green salads such as lettuce, romaine, endive, and cress and the citrous fruits which are oranges, lemons, grapefruit and limes.

These are called "protective foods" because they protect the body against certain diseases which will be described in the chapter on Nutrition. It is possible for a baby who nurses at the breast of a woman whose diet is poor in protective foods, to be so incompletely nourished as to be on the border line of one of these diseases, or even to develop the disease itself.

It becomes apparent, therefore, that although you did not have to "eat for two" before the baby came, you have to do so now in certain very important respects. For this reason it may be advisable for you to increase the nourishment provided by your three regular meals by taking a glass of milk, cocoa, or some beverage made of milk, during the morning and afternoon and before retiring.

The morning and afternoon lunches would better be taken about an hour and a half after breakfast and luncheon, respectively, in order not to spoil your appetite for the meals which follow. It is of considerable importance that you take your meals with clock-like regularity and enjoy them, as enjoyment promotes digestion; but at the same time you should guard against overeating for fear of causing indigestion, as this, you know, is almost sure to upset the baby. Rich and highly seasoned foods, in fact any articles of food or drink which might upset you, should be avoided for the same reason. Drink water freely but do not take alcohol nor strong tea or coffee without your doctor's permission.

Summing up the matter of your diet, we find that you should have light, nourishing, easily digestible food, consisting chiefly of cereals, creamed dishes, creamed soups, eggs, meat in moderation, salads and the fresh fruits and vegetables that ordinarily agree with you. Many doctors advise at least a quart of milk daily, in addition to that which is used in preparing the meals and an abundance of water to drink.

Bowels. Your bowels should move freely and regularly every day, but you should not take cathartics, or even enemata without your doctor's order. You probably will be able to establish the habit of a daily movement by taking exercise, eating bulky fruit and vegetables, drinking an abundance of water and regularly attempting to empty your bowels at the same time every day, preferably immediately after breakfast.

Rest and Exercise. You will not be likely to thrive, nor will the baby, unless you have adequate rest and sleep and take daily at least a moderate amount of exercise in the open air. You need eight hours sleep, out of twenty-four, in a room with the windows open, and as fatigue is bad for your milk it may be a good plan for you to lie down for a while every afternoon. Your exercise will, of course, have to be adjusted to your tastes, habits, circumstances and physical endurance, for it must always be stopped before you are tired. Walking is often the best form of exercise that the nursing mother can take and though as a rule she may engage in any mild sports that she enjoys, violent exercise is inadvisable because of the exhaustion that may follow.

Recreation. Part of the value of exercise lies in the pleasure and diversion which it offers, for as we have seen, a happy, contented frame of mind is practically indispensable to the production of good milk. In addition to some regular and enjoyable exercise, therefore, you need a certain amount of recreation and change of thought and environment. If life is monotonous and colorless, the average woman is almost sure to become irritable and depressed; to lose her poise and perspective; to worry and fret, and then, no matter what she eats nor how much she sleeps, her digestion will suffer, her milk will be affected and the baby will pay. This, of course, goes back to the question of the young mother's mental state and the condition of her nerves as determining factors in her ability to nurse the baby successfully.

Just here it is important to say a word of caution about this very question of your attitude of mind, particularly as it relates to your care of yourself.

It may be that one of the most difficult tasks you will have will be that of getting out of the habit of accepting the position that borders on being an invalid—of being a protected person who is thought about, cared for and considered at every turn. This has been your position for several months and the most natural result of it all is a tendency to cling, perhaps ever so little and even unconsciously, to this very pleasant state. It is not possible for anyone to reduce so broad and intangible a subject to a few definite words of advice. But think it over for yourself and try to strike that happiest of happy mediums that lies somewhere between the equally harmful courses of coddling yourself and of overdoing.

A good many doctors think that for the sake of giving the nursing mother an opportunity to go out, mingle with her friends, take in some music or a play, it is often a good plan to replace one breast feeding, sometime in the course of each day, with a bottle feeding. The freedom which this long interval between two nursings gives the mother for diversion and amusement, will often affect her general condition so favorably that the quality of her milk is definitely better than it otherwise would be and the baby is benefited as a result. This single supplementary feeding cannot be regarded lightly, however, for it must be prepared with the same cleanliness and accuracy as an entirely artificial diet, which will be described in the next chapter.

Weaning. One advantage in giving the baby a supplementary bottle once a day, is that it paves the way for weaning, when the time comes to make this change. Under ordinary conditions, the mother begins to wean her baby about the eighth or tenth month. Having started by replacing one breast feeding, daily, with a bottle feeding, she gradually increases the number of bottles given daily until the breast feedings are discontinued by the time the baby is eleven or twelve months old. There are exceptions to this general rule, of course, and under any conditions the weaning should always be directed by a doctor, for the baby may suffer seriously unless the change in food is skillfully made. If the mother's milk is satisfactory and the baby is doing well, it is often considered wise not to discontinue the breast feeding entirely, during the hot summer months even though the weaning falls due at this time.

It was formerly deemed advisable to wean the baby for any one of several reasons, but at present the only indications for this step which seem to be generally accepted by the medical profession, are: pulmonary tuberculosis, acute infectious diseases in the mother and pregnancy. Menstruation was long regarded as incompatible with satisfactory nursing, but it is now known that if the mother is taking proper care of herself and is in generally good condition, the impoverishing effect of menstruation upon the milk is usually for the duration of the periods only. It may be necessary to supplement the breast feeding with suitably modified cows' milk during menstruation, but the baby should be put to the breast regularly, just the same, for if the stimulation of the baby's suckling is discontinued, the temporary reduction in the amount of the milk secreted will probably become permanent.

The state of pregnancy, however, is different, for though some women nurse a baby satisfactorily for some months after becoming pregnant, it is not considered advisable to subject any woman to the combined strain of pregnancy and nursing. Moreover, the mother's milk is usually so impoverished during pregnancy that the nursing baby suffers in consequence.

Drying up the breasts used to be a great bugbear. Lotions, ointments and binders were employed and often a breast pump as well. Various drugs were given by mouth and the mother was more or less rigidly dieted. It is true that some of these measures are still employed and are followed by a disappearance of the milk. But at the same time, the breasts dry up quite as satisfactorily when none of these things are done, provided the baby does not nurse. It is not known what starts the secretion of milk in the mother's breasts, but certain it is that absence of the baby's suckling stops it.

If it is left to you to dry up your breasts, your safest course will be to do nothing beyond applying a supporting bandage, if your breasts are heavy enough to be uncomfortable, and keeping your nipples scrupulously clean. You may rely absolutely upon the fact that the baby's suckling is the most important stimulation in promoting the activity of the breasts and if this stimulation is not given, or is removed, the secretion of milk will invariably subside in the course of a few days. This is true whether the reason for drying up the breasts is that the baby is stillborn or has died, or a live baby's nursing is discontinued. It is true that the breasts may be swollen and very uncomfortable for a day or two, and in addition to a supporting bandage the doctor may order sedatives, but the discomfort subsides as the milk disappears.

Quite naturally you will not drink an extra amount of milk if you are drying up your breasts, but it probably will not be necessary to place any other restrictions upon your diet.

In thinking over the nursing period as a whole, we find that after all it is a fairly simple matter so to order one's life as to promote and maintain a satisfactory supply of milk. The milk thus produced is the ideal baby food and *there is no entirely adequate substitute*. Never forget that. It gives the baby enormously increased chances of living past babyhood and protects him from many diseases.

Quite evidently breast feeding is every baby's birthright and his mother is the only one who can deprive him of it.

CHAPTER X
THE MOTHER'S CARE OF HER BABY

"The mother is the natural guardian of her child; no other influence can compare with hers in its value in safeguarding infant life."—*Sir Arthur Newsholme.*

Before undertaking the care of the new baby, suppose we stop for a moment, and consider just what he represents; what he has been through; what struggles and dangers are ahead of him; what are the weaknesses of his equipment to meet these perils and what must be the character of your service to him if you are to do quite all in your power to help him safely over this hazardous period of early infancy.

At the time of birth, the baby makes the most complete and abrupt change in his surroundings and condition that he will make during his entire lifetime.

For nine months he has existed under ideal conditions; he has been safeguarded from injury; kept at the temperature which was best for him, and above all, has been furnished with exactly the proper amount and character of nourishment necessary for his growth and development. Suddenly he emerges from this completely protecting environment into a more or less hostile world, where he must assume the task of living, with a frail little body that in many respects is only imperfectly developed. And yet the baby must not only continue the bodily functions and activities that were begun during his intra-uterine life, but must develop certain functions which were imperfect and even establish others which were performed for him.

You will recall that while within the uterus, the baby received his nourishment and oxygen and gave up waste material through the placenta.

Accordingly, his organs of digestion, respiration and excretion are imperfectly developed at birth and are capable of functioning only within very narrow limits at first.

His respirations are usually established immediately after birth, when he cries vigorously, for his lungs are thereby filled with air. The other functions are established more gradually and the care of the baby must be such that the immature, unused organs will have their development promoted through activity and yet not be overtaxed.

The Baby's Condition at Birth. The newborn baby boy weighs from seven and a quarter to seven and a half pounds and is about twenty inches long, girl babies being perhaps a little smaller. His body is well rounded and his flesh firm. The skin is a deep pink, or even red, and is covered with the cheesy substance called vernix caseosa, which is likely to be thickly deposited over the back and in folds of the skin and creases, as in the thighs and under the arms. Some babies still have, when born, the fine downy hair on parts or all of the body, that they had before birth.

The head and abdomen are relatively large, the chest narrow and the limbs short. The legs are so markedly bowed that the soles of the baby's feet may nearly or quite face each other, but they finally assume a normal position. The bones are still soft and the entire body is, therefore, very flexible. Some of the bones which unite later in life and make the adult skeleton firm and rigid, are separate at birth.

Most newborn babies have faded blue eyes, the permanent color appearing gradually, but the amount and color of the hair varies greatly, some babies being bald, while others have abundant hair from the beginning.

The shape of the baby's head is often badly distorted at birth, being so long from chin to crown that the mother is deeply concerned. But you may rest quite assured that even though badly misshapen, your baby's head in the course of a few days will assume the lovely, rounded contour so characteristic of babyhood. The temporary deformity of the head is caused by a molding and overlapping of the bones of the skull as it is forced through the narrow part of the pelvis, the inlet, that we learned about in Chapter III. About the middle of the top of the head you will be able to feel a soft, diamond shaped spot and farther back another soft spot, smaller than the one in front and somewhat triangular in its outline. These soft places are openings between the bones of the skull and are called the *anterior* and *posterior fontanelles*. They always may be felt on the new baby's head.

Growth and Development. The physical progress which is made during the first year by average, normal babies who are satisfactorily nourished and cared for is fairly uniform and the average rate of this progress is somewhat as follows:

Weight. There is a loss in weight of 6 to 10 ounces during the first week of life, after which the baby usually gains from 4 to 8 ounces each week, during the first five months. From this time the gain is only about half as rapid, or at the rate of 2 to 4 ounces weekly. At six months, therefore, the average baby weighs from 15 to 16 pounds, or double the normal birth weight of 7½ pounds, and at twelve months he weighs from 20 to 22 pounds, or three times the average birth weight. Fig. 41 gives an idea of how the baby's weight drops during the first week and the rate of the normal weekly gain afterwards, during the first year.

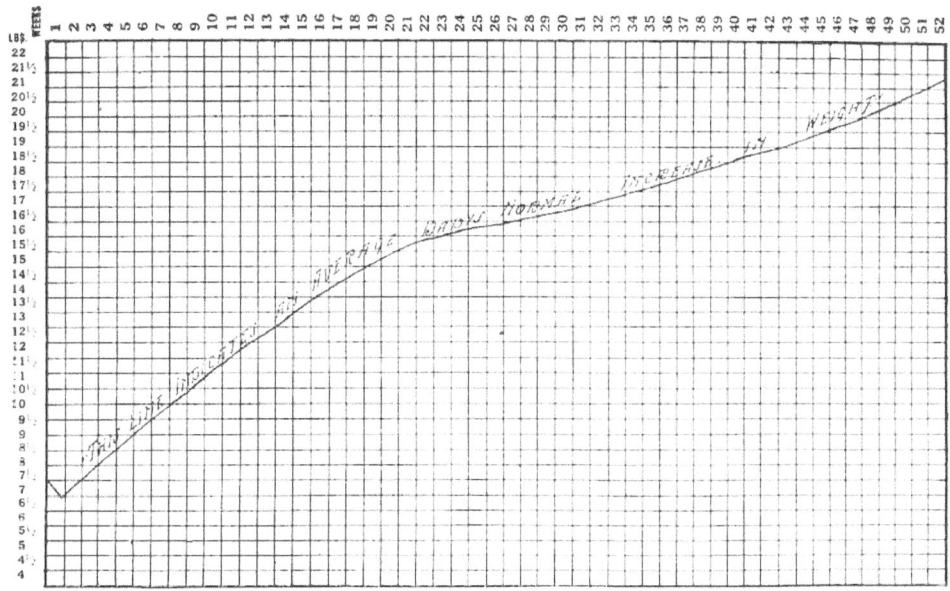

FIG. 41.—Baby's weight chart showing the usual loss during the first week and subsequent gain during the first year of life.

The weight is perhaps the most valuable single index to the baby's condition that we have, but at the same time it must be remembered that a baby whose food contains an excess of sugar or starch may be of normal weight, or over, but be incompletely nourished and very susceptible to infection, while other babies who are small and gain slowly are sometimes very well and vigorous. Moreover, quite commonly there are periods in the lives of entirely normal babies during which there is little or no gain in weight. This may occur during the period from the seventh to the tenth month, for example, or in very warm weather. But the doctor is likely to want to watch the baby's weight, for when studied in conjunction with other conditions it gives a certain amount of information about the baby's general state and progress.

Height. The height of the average baby at birth is about 20 inches, though boys may measure a little more and girls a little less; at six months it is about 25 inches and 28 or 29 inches at the end of a year.

Head and Chest. The circumferences of the head and chest are about the same at birth, the chest being possibly a little the smaller of the two. Both measure about 13½ inches, gradually increasing to about 16½ inches in six months and to 18 inches by the end of the first year.

Fontanelles. The posterior fontanelle, the one at the crown of the head, usually closes in six or eight weeks but the larger, anterior fontanelle is not entirely closed until the baby is about eighteen or twenty months old.

Teeth. Although it occasionally happens that a baby has one or two teeth at birth, the average infant has none until the sixth or seventh month, when the two lower, central incisors appear. After a pause of a few weeks the two upper, central incisors come through, followed by the two lateral incisors in the upper jaw. At the end of the first year, therefore, the average baby has six teeth, or eight if the lower lateral incisors have appeared by the first birthday, as they sometimes do. This is the usual course of dentition, during the first year, as shown in Fig. 42, but there are wide variations among entirely well and normal babies, the first tooth sometimes not appearing before the tenth, eleventh or even twelfth month. As a rule, however, an entire lack of teeth by the time the baby is a year old is regarded as an evidence of faulty nutrition.

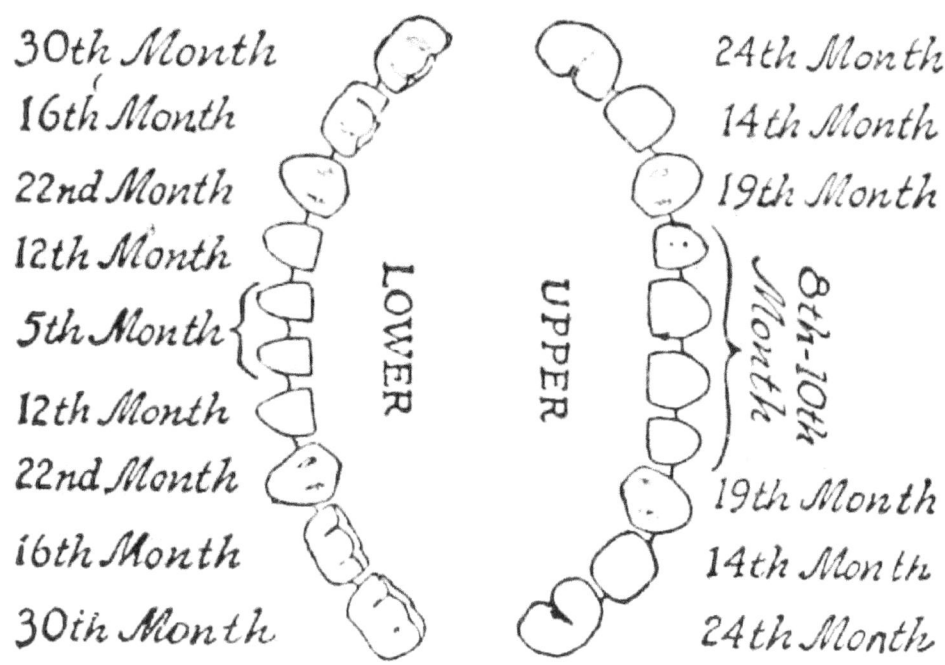

Fig. 42.—Diagram showing first, or "milk," teeth and the ages at which they usually appear.

The baby who is properly fed and cared for, cuts his teeth with little or no trouble, in spite of the widely current but seriously mistaken belief that a teething baby is a sick baby. We have no way of estimating the number of babies who die, needlessly, as a result of this dangerous conviction, for if the baby is sick while teething, the trouble is all too often accepted as a normal occurrence and is not given the attention it needs until too late. Frail, delicate babies may have convulsions each time that a tooth is cut and if a baby is having digestive trouble, this is likely to grow worse while he is teething. But cutting teeth is a normal process and the healthy, properly fed baby suffers little or no inconvenience while it is in progress.

Stools and Urine. During the first two or three days the stools are of dark green, tarry material called meconium. In the course of two or three days they begin to grow lighter and shortly the normal stools appear, these being bright yellow in color, of a smooth, pasty consistency and having a characteristic odor. During the first month or six weeks the baby's bowels may move three or four times daily, but after this they usually move but once or twice in the course of twenty-four hours. As the nourishment is increased, the stools grow somewhat darker and firmer and finally become formed.

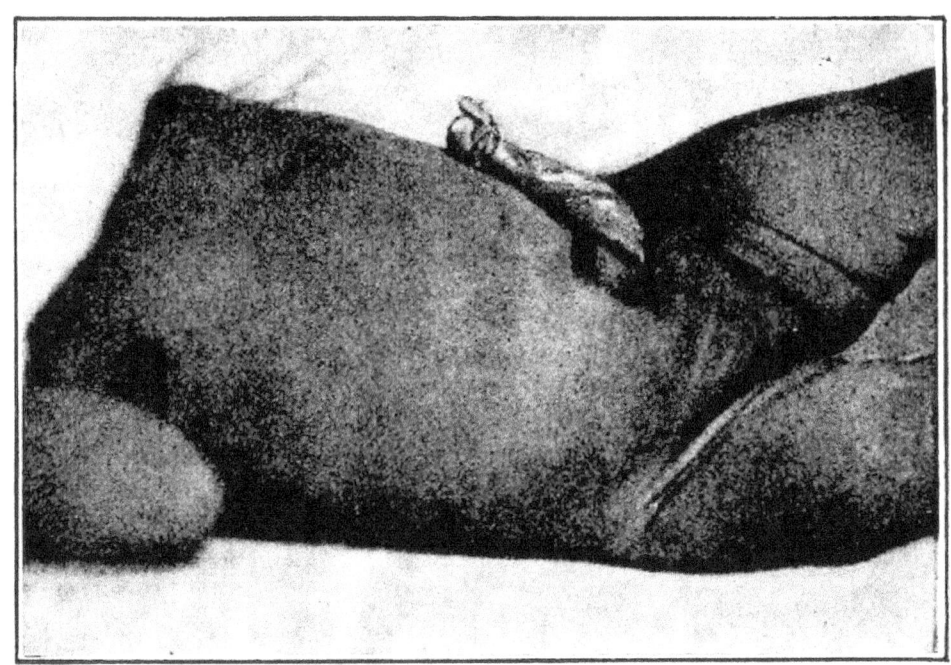

Fig. 43.—Appearance of cord immediately after birth.

The newborn baby's bladder usually contains urine and this may be passed immediately after birth or not until several hours later. After the first urination the bladder may be emptied five or six times a day or oftener.

The Cord. Within a few days after birth the stump of the umbilical cord that is attached to the baby's navel, begins to shrivel and turn black and a red line appears where the cord joins the abdomen. By the eighth or tenth day, as a rule, the cord has shrunken to a dry, black string, when it drops off and leaves an ulcer or small red area which heals entirely in the course of a few days. Figs. 43, 44, 45 and 46 show these progressive changes.

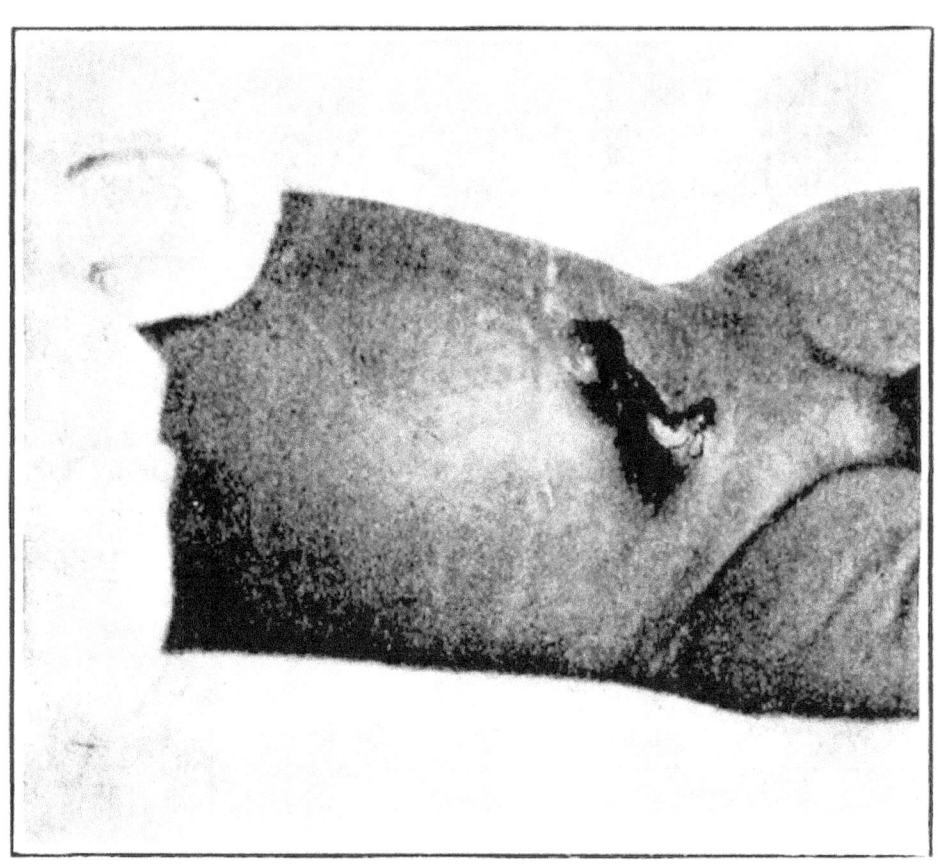

Fig. 44.—Appearance of cord four days after birth.

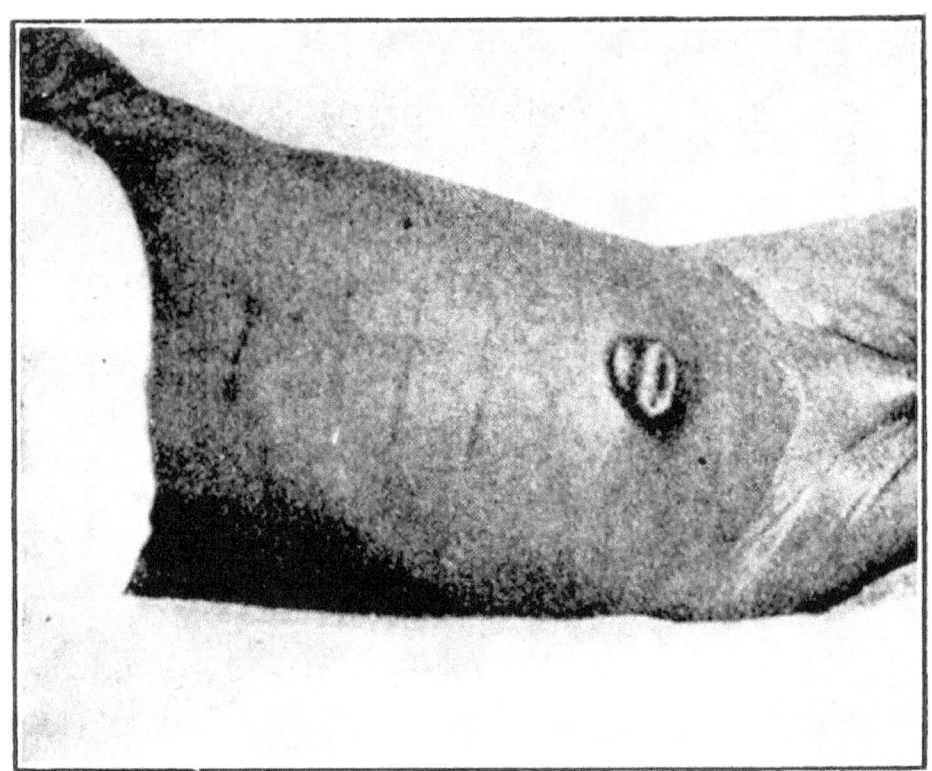

Fig. 45.—Appearance of navel immediately after cord has dropped off.

Skin. The soft, downy hair that may be remaining on the surface of the body usually disappears by the end of the first week and there is often a scaling of the skin which lasts for two or three weeks, while a delicate pink tint replaces the deeper color of the skin in the course of ten days or two weeks. The baby does not perspire until after the first month, ordinarily, when a very slight perspiration begins, gradually increasing until by the time the baby is a few months old he is perspiring freely.

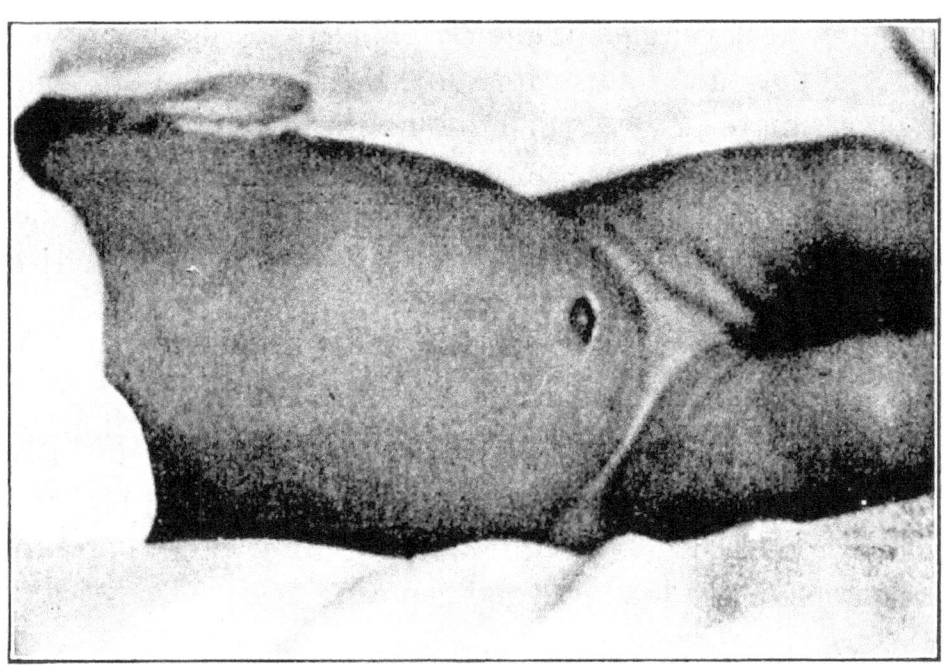

Fig. 46.—Appearance of a normal, well healed navel.

Tears. There are no tears at birth and opinions differ as to whether they appear in the course of two or three weeks or three or four months. The absence of tears is one reason for bathing the baby's eyes so carefully during the early days and weeks, for if dust or other foreign material gets into the eyes it is not washed out by tears as it is after their flow is established.

General Behavior. During the first few weeks the average baby sleeps most of the time; that is, from 19 to 21 hours daily. He gradually sleeps less, as the special senses develop and will sometimes lie quietly for an hour or more with his eyes open, sleeping only 16 or 18 hours, daily, at six months and 14 to 16 hours at the end of a year.

The baby begins to make noises and "coo" at about two months and to utter various vowel sounds when about six months old. By the end of a year these indefinite noises and sounds become distinct words. At about the fourth month he grasps at objects and smiles, and very soon even laughs. He holds up his head at about the third or fourth month; sits up and also begins to creep at six or seven months, while sometime between the ninth and twelfth months he will stand while holding on to something secure and begin to walk with assistance.

These degrees of development at different ages are not to be taken as the only measure of normal progress, for some well babies mature more rapidly and many others more slowly than at the rate which is found to be average. In addition to these fairly specific evidences of the baby's condition and progress, such as weight, height, strength and muscular development, there are other and less definite indications of his well-being which should be taken into account.

The baby who is well and is being properly fed in all respects, will have good color; his flesh will be firm; he will take his nourishment with a certain amount of eagerness and seem satisfied afterwards. He will sleep for two or three hours after each feeding; will sleep quietly at night and while awake, unless he is wet or uncomfortable for some other good reason, he will seem contented, good-natured and happy.

You have seen how the average, well baby grows and develops, provided he is given proper care. I want you now to have just a glimpse of the other side of the question, so that you may realize what happens to the unfortunate little citizens who are not given such care. This glimpse will make you realize more than ever, how worth while are all of the precautions that you take for your baby.

It is estimated that out of every 1000 babies born alive, in this country, 40 die during the first month of life, and that more than as many again, or about 85 all told, perish before reaching the first birthday.

So hazardous is this period of early infancy, in the United States, that our annual loss of baby life is between seven and eight times as great as was the yearly loss of our young men in the war, for upwards of 200,000 babies less than a year old die each year. That the first month is more dangerous than any which follow is shown by the fact that about 100,000 of these baby deaths occur during the first four weeks of life. The tragedy of these figures is made darker by the fact that at least half of the babies who are lost die from preventable causes. In other words, they die from lack of proper care.

That is the point of this for you. These babies die, not by an act of Providence, but from lack of care—not the difficult, complicated care needed by sick babies but just the everyday care which any mother may give—the care that keeps well babies well.

That is what you are going to do—keep your well baby well. And you are going to be surprised to find how easy it is, after all, to say nothing of the pleasure of it, for the thing very nearly sums itself up into feeding your baby as the doctor orders and keeping him clean in every particular. Bear these two factors in mind for errors in feeding and lack of cleanliness are the underlying causes of the vast majority of baby ills.

You will often feel a little like Alice in Wonderland, who found, one time, that she had to keep running very fast to stay where she was, for you will not be able to relax in a single detail of your baby's care if you are to keep him well. With him, as with you, or anyone else, the satisfactory use of even ideal food is largely dependent upon the general condition and mode of living, and we find accordingly, that the question of keeping the baby well finally resolves itself into the following common sense requirements:

1. Proper food.
2. Fresh air.
3. Regularity in the daily routine care.
4. Cleanliness of food, clothing and surroundings.
5. Preservation of an even body temperature.
6. Adequate rest and sleep.
7. Periodic consultations with your doctor.

Carve these principles into the tablets of your brain and you cannot fail to give your baby the kind of care that is literally life-saving. I am going to describe the tiny, intimate details of this care, for I think this will help you, in the beginning at least, but if you will keep these fundamentals in mind and use good common sense you really need not read another word about baby care, for they give it all in a nutshell.

Let me warn you emphatically against making the very serious mistake of acting upon the advice of friends or relatives, no matter how many children they have had. These counselors are just as dangerous for babies as they are for expectant mothers, so beware of them!

"Is it not preposterous," says Herbert Spencer, "that the fate of a new generation should be left to the chance of unreasoning custom, impulse, fancy, joined with the suggestions of ignorant nurses and the prejudiced counsel of grandmothers? To tens of thousands that are killed, add hundreds of thousands that survive with feeble constitutions, and millions that grow up with constitutions not so strong as they should be, and you have some idea of the curse inflicted on their offspring by parents ignorant of the laws of life."

It is a very wise precaution to have your doctor see the baby every week or ten days during the first three months and once a month during the remainder of the year. Not because he is fragile or ill. Not at all. You consult your doctor in order to be sure that you are *keeping your baby well*.

Did you ever hear of the Chinese custom of paying the doctor as long as one is well, but not paying for attention during illness? It isn't so very heathenish—that idea of paying for the skillful care that will prevent illness.

In addition to taking the general precaution of seeing your doctor periodically, about the baby, be sure to consult him about anything that you do not understand or about any new condition that arises. You will find any number of persons who are ready and eager to advise you, but your doctor is the only one whose advice it is safe for you to follow.

The Daily Schedule. The importance of regularity in the daily routine of the baby's care cannot be stressed too often nor too insistently. No matter how well he is nursed in other respects, nor how skillfully the doctor directs his care, the baby cannot be expected to progress satisfactorily if his life is not absolutely regular.

Begin by arranging a daily program for the feedings, fresh air, bath, sleep and exercise and then allow nothing to interfere with your carrying it out.

The hours for the nursings, which vary with different doctors, will constitute the greater part of this daily schedule. For a baby on four hour feedings, for example, some such program as the following may be arranged, while for a baby on a three hour schedule a slightly different program may be arranged.

	6	a.m.	Feeding.
	8	a.m.	Orange juice (when ordered).
	9	a.m.	Bath.
	10	a.m.	Feeding.
10:30 to	2	p.m.	Out of doors.
	2	p.m.	Feeding.
2:30 to	4	p.m.	Out of doors.
	4	p.m.	Orange juice (when ordered).
4 to	5:30	p.m.	Indoor airing and exercises (when ordered).
	5:30	p.m.	Preparation for the night.
	6 p.m.		Feeding.
	10 p.m.		Feeding.
	2 a.m.		Feeding (when ordered).

YOUR BABY'S FOOD

Proper feeding is probably the most decisive single factor in the routine care of the baby.

In order that the food shall be satisfactory, it must be not only suitable in composition for the individual baby, but it must be clean, fresh and at the right temperature; given in suitable amounts and at suitable intervals; it must be given properly—not too fast nor too slowly and it must be given under favorable conditions. Moreover, as has been stated, the baby, himself, must be kept in a general condition which will promote the digestion and assimilation of the food that is given to him. Fresh air, suitable clothing, an even body temperature, gentle handling, proper bathing, regular sleep, freedom from excitement, fatigue, and irritation all promote the baby's ability to use his food to advantage. Reverse conditions all work against it. Accordingly, the actual value of the baby's food to him will be largely dependent upon the care that you give him.

There are three methods of nourishing the baby: by breast feeding, by artificial feeding and by a combination of the two, termed mixed or supplementary feeding.

Breast Feeding. From all standpoints, maternal nursing, under normal conditions, is the most satisfactory method of nourishing a baby. If the breast milk is suitable it meets all of the baby's requirements and the proportion and character of its constituents are exactly suited to his digestive powers. In order for maternal nursing to be entirely satisfactory, the condition of both mother and baby must be favorable. The preparation and care of the mother have been described: her general condition and state of nutrition; the care and condition of her nipples, flat or retracted nipples being· brought out if possible, and if not, the nursing facilitated by the use of a shield. As to the baby, if his diaper is wet or soiled, it should be changed before he is put to the breast, partly to make him comfortable and partly to avoid disturbing him for this after his feeding; and his mouth is gently swabbed with boric-soaked cotton, if your doctor so orders.[2]

2. Boracic acid solution is made by adding one teaspoonful of the crystals to one cup (half-pint) of boiling water.

Although nursing is an instinct, the baby may have to learn how to nurse or to acquire the habit, this being one reason for putting him to the breast during those first two or three days when he obtains little or no actual food, as was explained in Chapter IX. As he expresses the milk by squeezing and suction made possible only when the nipple is well back in his mouth, he must take into his mouth practically the entire colored area which surrounds the nipple. To do this he lies in the curve of his mother's arm as she turns slightly to one side, and holds her breast away from his nostrils in order that he may breathe freely.

Sometimes, even when other conditions are favorable, the baby is unable to nurse because of some physical disability. He may be too feeble, may have a cleft palate or find suckling painful because of an injury to the mucous membrane which occurred when his mouth was wiped out just after birth. The manner in which the baby nurses, therefore, may be significant and should be described to the doctor if there is any difficulty.

When the baby has finished nursing he should be taken up very gently, held upright against the shoulder for a moment or two, to help him bring up gas if he has any, and then placed in his crib and left to sleep. If he is nursing satisfactorily, he will be sleepy and contented afterwards and will sleep for two or three hours; he will seem generally good-humored and comfortable while awake; he will have good color; gain weight steadily and have two or three normal bowel movements daily. The normal stool in breast-fed babies is bright yellow, smooth and has no evidences of undigested food.

If the baby is not being adequately nourished, he will present exactly the opposite picture, in some or all of these respects. He will be unwilling to stop nursing after the normal length of time and will give evidence of being not satisfied when taken from the breast. He may be listless and fretful and sleep badly. He will not gain weight as he should and he may vomit or have colic after nursing.

To ascertain whether or not such a baby is getting enough milk it is customary to weigh him, without undressing him, before and after each nursing. Each fluid ounce of milk will increase his weight one ounce. If the baby is not obtaining a normal amount of milk at each nursing, he is often given enough modified milk after each meal to supply the shortage, but at the same time an effort is made to increase the supply of breast milk by improving the mother's personal hygiene, as described in Chapter IX.

The amount which the baby needs at each feeding varies, not only according to his weight and age, but also according to his vigor and activity and therefore must be estimated for each baby. A very general estimate of the amount taken by the average, well baby at each feeding, is about as follows:

First week	1½ to 2½	ounces
Second and third week	2 to 4	ounces
Fourth to ninth week	3 to 4½	ounces
Tenth week to fifth month	3½ to 5	ounces
Fifth to seventh month	4½ to 6½	ounces
Seventh to twelfth month	6½ to 9	ounces

Artificial Feeding. There is no entirely adequate substitute for satisfactory maternal nursing, and any other food that is given to the young baby is at best a makeshift. Considering the baby's delicacy, therefore, and his urgent needs, no pains should be spared to make any artificial food that is given to him, as satisfactory as possible. And no matter what it costs, he should have only the freshest, cleanest and purest milk that can be bought.

In preparing and giving artificial food it must be borne in mind that normal breast milk has the following characteristics:

1. It is exactly right in quantity, quality and proportion.
2. It is fresh, clean and sweet.
3. It is free from bacteria.
4. It tends to protect the baby from infection.
5. It definitely protects him from certain nutritional diseases.

Cows' milk, suitably modified, is apparently the best available substitute for mother's milk, but it must first meet certain requirements and then be handled with scrupulous cleanliness and care, if it is to be satisfactory.

The requirements are that the milk shall be:

1. Whole milk. It must not be altered by the removal of cream nor the addition of such preservatives as salicylic acid, formaldehyde or boracic acid.
2. Its composition must not vary greatly from day to day.
3. It must be clean and free from disease germs; other organisms should not be present in excessive numbers.
4. It must be fresh; less than 24 hours old when it is delivered.

All of this means that the milk must come from a herd of healthy, tuberculin-tested cows. The milk from a single cow may vary markedly from day to day but that from several cows is nearly constant. The stables and the cows must be kept clean, the udders carefully washed before each milking; the milkers themselves must wear freshly washed clothing, scrub their hands thoroughly and milk into sterile receptacles; the milk must be immediately covered and cooled to a temperature of 45° F. or 50° F. and kept there.

Milk produced under such conditions is usually described as "certified milk" and is often prescribed as infant food without being pasteurized or sterilized. But if there is any doubt about the source of the milk and the method of its handling, it should be strained into a clean receptacle through filter paper or a thick layer of absorbent cotton and subsequently boiled or pasteurized.

Whether certified or not, the milk should invariably be placed in the refrigerator, or some other place which has a temperature of 50° F., as soon as it is received, and *it must be kept cool and clean.*

Keeping milk cool means keeping it at a temperature of 50° F. Keeping it clean implies cleanliness not alone of the milk itself but of your hands and the utensils that you use as well as the destruction of disease germs by pasteurization or sterilization. Among the germs which are likely to be present in infected milk are those that cause diarrhea, sore throats, typhoid fever, diphtheria and scarlet fever.

When the doctor makes out the formula for the baby's milk, he will adjust the proportions of the different ingredients to the baby's immediate needs and digestive powers. But his careful estimations will be set at naught unless you are absolutely *accurate* in preparing and giving the milk. Your invariable responsibility in connection with the baby's milk, therefore, is to keep it *cool* and *clean* and be *accurate*.

You will appreciate the necessity for modifying cows' milk before giving it to your baby if you will note the differences between mother's milk and cows' milk as indicated by the following table and consider, too, why Nature has made these differences:

	Mother's Milk			*Cows' Milk*		
Fats	3.5 to	4.	per cent	3.5 to	4.	per cent
Sugar	6.5 to	7.5	per cent	4.5 to	4.75	per cent
Proteins	1. to	1.5	per cent	3.5 to	4.	per cent
Salts		.2	per cent	.7 to	.75	per cent
Water	87. to	88.	per cent		87.	per cent

The various tissues of the body and the bony skeleton are built by the proteins and salt. Accordingly Nature supplies these in greater abundance to the baby calf, who grows so fast as to double his birth weight in about forty-seven days, than to the baby boy who scarcely doubles his birth weight within 180 days. The calf begins life with a physical need for the large amount of proteins and salts which are present in cows' milk and with digestive organs that can cope with them, but the baby needs less, can digest less and, therefore, should be given less. There are of course, other and finer differences between the two milks and an attempt is sometimes make to meet these. For example, mother's milk is slightly alkaline and cows' milk slightly acid and the curd of cows' milk is larger, tougher and harder to digest than that formed by mother's milk. Some doctors add lime water to cows' milk, before giving it to the baby, to make it alkaline and have the curd made softer, finer and more digestible by boiling.

Articles Needed in Preparing the Baby's Food. A complete equipment for preparing and giving the baby's milk should be assembled, kept in a clean place, separate from utensils in general use, and never put to any other service. A satisfactory outfit for this purpose comprises the following articles:

One dozen graduated nursing bottles.
One dozen nipples.

Clean, new corks or a package of sterile, non-absorbent cotton for stoppers.
Bottle brush.
Covered kettle, capacity one gallon, for boiling bottles and possibly pasteurizing milk.
Pasteurizer or wire bottle rack.
Small kettle, about one quart size.
Graduated pint or quart measuring glass.
Pitcher, two-quart size.
Long-handled spoon for mixing.
Funnel.
Measuring spoons—table and tea sizes.
Double boiler.
Thermometer which will register at least 212° F.
Cream dipper (if ordered).
Two small covered jars for sterile and used nipples.
Sugar (lactose, maltose or cane sugar according to orders).
Lime water (if ordered).

Utensils of enamel or aluminum ware are probably the most satisfactory ones to use as they are easily kept clean, while bottles with wide mouths and curved bottoms and inner surfaces can be thoroughly washed more easily than those with small necks and sharp corners. Nipples that can be turned inside out to be washed should be selected as it is almost impossible to clean thoroughly those with tubes or narrow necks. New bottles will be rendered less breakable if placed in cold water, which is gradually heated, allowed to boil for half an hour and cooled before the bottles are removed.

The bottles should be rinsed with cold water after each feeding and then carefully washed and scrubbed with the bottle brush in hot soapsuds or borax water, containing two tablespoonfuls to the pint. They may be kept full of water while not in use or rinsed with hot water and stood upside down until they are all boiled on the following morning, preparatory to being filled with the freshly prepared milk. The baby's bottles should never be washed in dishwater nor dried on a towel. The nipples should be rinsed in cold water, turned inside out and scrubbed with a brush, in hot soapsuds or borax water; rinsed and placed in a jar ready to be boiled with the bottles.

Preparing the Milk. The full quantity of milk which the baby will take in the course of twenty-four hours is prepared at one time and the prescribed amount for each feeding poured into as many separate bottles as there will be feedings.

You should begin by assembling on a table everything that you will use in preparing the milk formula, as the nurse has in Fig. 47. Boil for five minutes all of the articles that will come in contact with the milk, including the full number of bottles and nipples and the jars in which the nipples are kept; remove them with the long-handled spoon without touching the edges or inner surfaces, dropping the nipples into one of the sterile jars.

Wash the mouth of the milk bottle before removing the cap and pour the amount which the formula calls for into the sterile pitcher. To this is added the sterile water in which the sugar has been dissolved in the measuring glass and then the potato or barley water, the lime water or soda solution as ordered. This mixture is thoroughly stirred and the amount for one feeding at a time, measured in the measuring glass and poured into the specified number of bottles, which are then stoppered.

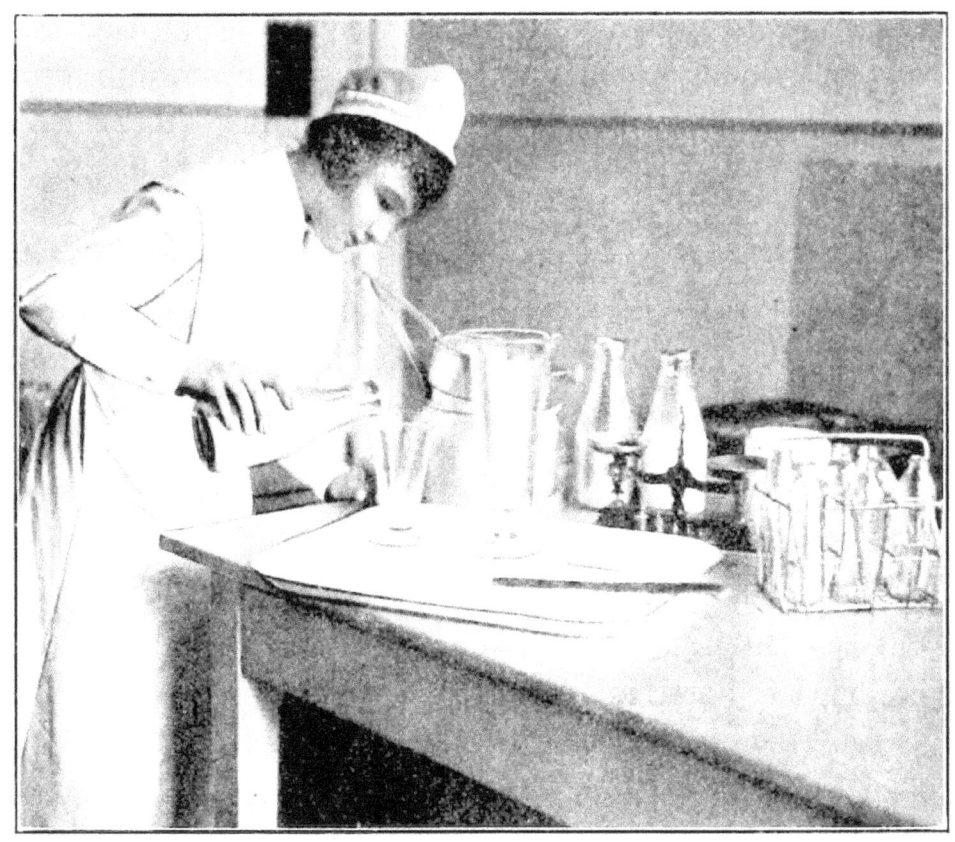

Fig. 47.—Preparing the baby's milk. (From a photograph taken at Johns Hopkins Hospital.)

If certified milk is used for the milk mixture it is often given to the baby without being pasteurized, in which case the bottles are placed in the refrigerator as soon as they are filled and stoppered. Very frequently, however, the milk is sterilized or pasteurized. You will feel surer of keeping the mouths of the bottles clean if you cover them with squares of gauze or muslin before they are sterilized, holding the caps in place with tapes or rubber bands.

Pasteurization as applied to infant feeding consists of heating the milk to 140–165° F. and keeping it at that temperature for 20 to 30 minutes.

There are many excellent pasteurizers for home use on the market, but entirely satisfactory results may be obtained by improvising one from the wire bottle rack seen in Fig. 47, and the large kettle already provided. One method is to place the rack, containing the bottles, in the kettle which is filled with cold water to a level a little above the top of the milk in the bottles, and allow the water to come to the boiling point. The kettle is removed from the fire, covered tightly and the bottles allowed to stand in the hot water for twenty minutes. Cold water is then run into the kettle to cool the milk gradually and avoid breaking the bottles, after which they are placed in the refrigerator, well or spring-house and kept at a temperature of 50° F. until they are taken out, one at a time, for feedings. If a wire rack is not available the bottles may be stood on a saucer or a thick pad of folded newspapers in the bottom of the kettle.

Pasteurization does not destroy all germs that may be in the milk, but it kills the more important ones and apparently impairs the nutritive and protective properties of the milk less than boiling. However, pasteurized milk must be kept cold and must be used within twenty-four hours, for the aging of milk is quite as undesirable as souring.

Scalding is another method of destroying germs in milk. The milk is placed in an open vessel and the temperature raised to about 180° F., or until bubbles appear around the edge and the milk steams in the center, after which it is cooled and kept at a temperature of 50° F.

Many doctors prefer to have the baby's milk boiled, since boiling insures absolute sterilization and also renders the curd more digestible. Other changes are produced by boiling, however, which make it important to add orange juice and cod-liver oil to the baby's diet at an early date, as will be explained in the next chapter.

Milk may be boiled directly over the flame for a time varying from three to forty-five minutes, or it may be placed in a double boiler, the water in the lower receptacle being cold, and allowed to remain until the water has boiled from six to forty-five minutes.

When milk is boiled or scalded, the other ingredients are added beforehand, as a rule, after which it is measured and poured into the bottles. Or the milk mixture may be poured into the bottles as for pasteurization and the bottles kept in the actively boiling water for any desired length of time.

All of these points, however, are definitely specified by the doctor.

Giving the Baby His Bottle. At feeding time, the bottle should be taken from the refrigerator, the stopper removed and a sterile nipple taken up by the margin and put on the bottle without touching the mouthpiece. The milk is brought to a temperature of about 100° F. by standing the bottle in a deep cup or kettle of warm water and placing it on the fire. The temperature of the milk may be tested by dropping a few drops on the inner side of the wrist or forearm where it should feel warm but not hot. This dropping will also indicate if the hole in the nipple is of the proper size to allow the milk to drop rapidly in clean drops but not to pour. If the hole is too small, the drops will be small and infrequent and the baby will be obliged to work too hard to obtain it; while if the hole is too large the baby will feed too rapidly and may have colic as a result. If the hole is too large the nipple will have to be discarded; if too small or if there is no hole, one of the proper size may be made by piercing the nipple with a heated darning needle or small steel knitting needle.

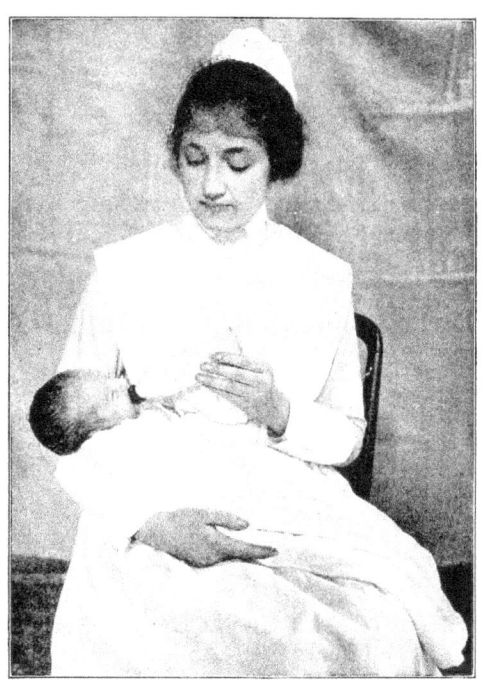

FIG. 48.—Proper position in which to hold baby and bottle during feeding.

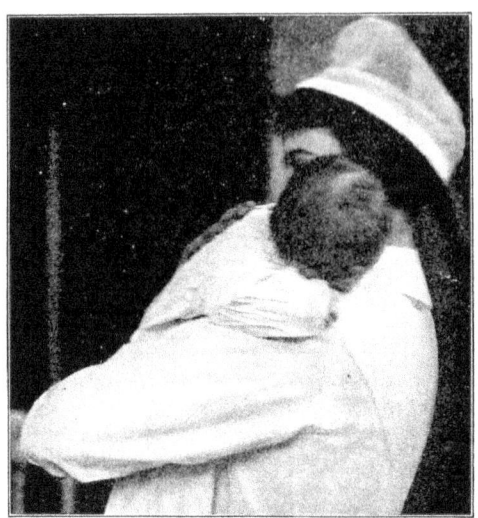

Fig. 49.—Holding the baby upright immediately after feeding, and gently patting his back to help him bring up air in order to prevent colic.

The baby's diaper should be changed if it is soiled or wet before he is given the bottle and he should be held comfortably on your arm, in a reclining position, while you hold the bottle with your free hand as shown by the nurse in Fig. 48. The bottle should be inclined sufficiently to keep the neck full of milk; otherwise the baby may draw in air as he nurses. He should be kept awake while feeding but he should be allowed to pause every three or four minutes in order not to take his milk too rapidly. Not less than ten nor more than twenty minutes is devoted to a feeding, as a rule, and if the baby refuses a part of his milk, it should be thrown away; never warmed over for another time.

After being fed, the baby should be held upright against your shoulder for a moment or two, as in Fig. 49, and ever so gently patted on the back to help bring up any air which he may have swallowed. He should on no account be rocked nor played with after taking the bottle, but should be placed gently in his crib, warm and dry and left alone to sleep. Turning him or moving him about even to the extent of changing his diaper at this time may cause vomiting.

The evidences of satisfactory and unsatisfactory feeding in the bottle-fed baby are about the same as in the baby who is fed at the breast, except that the gain in weight on artificial food may be a little slower and less steady than on maternal nursing; the stools have a characteristic sour odor; are a little lighter in color and may contain white lumps of undigested fat; are usually dryer than in breast feeding and may be formed, in even a very young baby.

Many doctors feel that all babies, whether breast-fed or on the bottle, require a certain amount of cool boiled water to drink between feedings. A small amount is given at first and gradually increased according to the doctor's instructions, and it may be given from a bottle, a medicine dropper or poured slowly from the tip of a teaspoon.

I feel sure that you have realized, long before this, that the entire question of planning the baby's food is such an important and complicated matter that it cannot with safety to the baby be undertaken by any one but your doctor. Unexpected situations do arise, however, when the doctor is not within immediate reach and the mother has to plan the baby's food, temporarily, to the best of her ability.

Should you find yourself in such an emergency, you will find help in the milk formulas contained in a pamphlet issued by the American Medical Association, remembering that they are intended for the average, normal baby and are not necessarily suitable for all babies. A large, vigorous baby may need more food and a small, frail baby have to take less than the amounts specified in the following directions:[3]

[3]. From "Save The Babies" by Dr. L. Emmet Holt and Dr. H. K. L. Shaw. Copied by courtesy of The American Medical Association.

"The simplest plan is to use whole milk (from a shaken bottle) which is to be diluted according to the child's age and digestion.

"Beginning on the third day, the average baby should be given 3 ounces of milk daily, diluted with seven ounces of water. To this should be added one tablespoonful of lime water and 2 level teaspoonfuls of sugar. This should be given in 7 feedings.

"At one week, the average child requires 5 ounces of milk daily, which should be diluted with 10 ounces of water. To this should be added 1½ even tablespoonfuls of sugar and one ounce of lime water. This should be given in 7 feedings.

"The milk should be increased by ½ ounce about every 4 days.

"The water should be increased by ½ ounce about every 8 days.

"At 3 months the average child requires 16 ounces of milk daily, which should be diluted with 16 ounces of water. To this should be added 3 tablespoonfuls of sugar and 2 ounces of lime water. This should be given in 6 feedings.

"The milk should be increased by ½ ounce about every 6 days.

"The water should be reduced by ½ ounce about every 2 weeks.

"At 6 months the average child requires 24 ounces of milk daily, which should be diluted with 12 ounces of water. To this should be added 2 ounces of lime water and 3 even tablespoonfuls of sugar. This should be given in 5 feedings.

"The amount of milk should be increased by ½ ounce every week.

"The milk should be increased only if the child is hungry and digesting his food well. It should not be increased unless he is hungry, nor if he is suffering from indigestion even though he seems hungry.

"At 9 months, the average child requires 30 ounces of milk daily, which should be diluted with 10 ounces of water. To this should be added 2 even tablespoonfuls of sugar and 2 ounces of lime water. This should be given in 5 feedings.

"The sugar added may be milk sugar or, if this cannot be obtained, cane (granulated) sugar or maltose (malt sugar).

"At first plain water should be used to dilute the milk.

"At 3 months, sometimes earlier, weak barley water may be used in the place of plain water; it is made with ½ level tablespoonful of barley flour to 16 ounces of water and cooked 20 minutes.

"At 6 months the barley flour may be increased to 1½ even tablespoonfuls, cooked in the 12 ounces of water.

"At 9 months, the barley flour may be increased to 3 level tablespoonfuls, cooked in the 10 ounces of water.

"A very large baby may require a little more milk than that allowed in these formulas. A small delicate baby will require less than the milk allowed in the formulas."

These formulas may be tabulated as shown on p. 177.

Mixed Feeding. Under some conditions the breast-fed baby is given also a certain amount of modified milk, and this combination of natural and artificial feeding is termed mixed or supplementary feeding.

A deficiency in the breast milk, ascertained by weighing the baby before and after each nursing, may be supplied by following each nursing with a bottle feeding; or for some reason, one or two breast feedings, in the course of the day are sometimes replaced by entire bottle feedings. In any case the milk mixture to be used as supplementary feeding is prepared with exactly the same painstaking care as is the milk for entire artificial feeding.

If supplementary food is given because of an inadequate supply of breast milk, it is of great importance that the baby be put to the breast regularly, no matter how little food he obtains, for his suckling is the best possible means of stimulating the breasts to secrete more milk, and of equal importance is the fact that they will tend to dry up if the baby nurses less than about five times in twenty-four hours. Moreover, even a little breast milk is valuable to him and he should have the benefit of all there is to be had.

Age	Milk	Water	Barley Water	Lime Water	Sugar	No. of feedings	Hours	
							Day	Night
3–7 days	3 ozs.	7 ozs.		½ ozs.	2 teaspoons	7	6– 9– 12– 3–6	10–2
2d week	5 "	10 "		1 "	1½ tablespoons	7	6– 9– 12– 3–6	10–2
3d "	6 "	10½ "		1 "	1½ "	7	6– 9– 12– 3–6	10–2
1 month	7 "	11 "		1 "	2 "	7	6– 9– 12– 3–6	10–2
2 "	11 "	13 "		1½ "	2½ "	7	6– 9– 12– 3–6	10–2
3 "	16 "		16 ozs.	2 "	3 "	7	6– 9– 12– 3–6	10–2
4 "	19 "		15 "	2 "	3 "	6	6– 9– 12– 3–6	10
5 "	21½ "		14 "	2 "	3 "	6	6– 9– 12– 3–6	10
6 "	24 "		12 "	2 "	3 "	5	6– 10– 2–6	10
7 "	26 "		12 "	2 "	3 "	5	6– 10– 2–6	10
8 "	28 "		11 "	2 "	2½ "	5	6– 10– 2–6	10
9 "	30 "		10 "	2 "	2 "	5	6– 10– 2–6	10

An entire bottle feeding is sometimes given to a baby who is nursing satisfactorily at the breast, in order to give his mother an opportunity to take longer outings than are possible between the regular nursings. And sometimes it is to the mother's advantage, and therefore to the baby's, to give him a bottle during the night and thus allow her to sleep undisturbed.

COMMERCIAL BABY FOODS

Since the baby's nourishment is prescribed by the doctor, you have no reason to concern yourself with the various proprietary baby foods and canned and powdered milks that are so persuasively advertised to young mothers. And I earnestly hope that by the time you finish this little book, no one will be able to make you believe that any of these foods is likely to be satisfactory if used as a sole article of diet throughout the bottle-feeding period.

Unquestionably there are many times and circumstances when the temporary or supplementary use of a prepared infant food or canned or powdered milk is advantageous.

In some cases of intestinal disturbance a proprietary food may be a great boon, or while the mother is traveling and is unable to have freshly prepared milk formulas supplied to her along the way. These foods may be valuable, also, during the summer, while one stays at a hotel or boarding house where the freshness, cleanliness or purity of the milk are uncertain, or during a sudden shortage of fresh milk, as may occur during a strike or severe storm when transportation is interrupted. But you should not use a prepared infant food for any length of time without your doctor's order.

If you are confronted with the necessity of choosing a prepared food, for temporary use, you may be guided by considering the general objects and principles of baby feeding and the character of the various foods at your disposal.

The proprietary foods may be divided into two general groups: one kind contains milk powder and is usually added to water, while the other consists largely of sugar and starch and is added to fresh milk before being given to the baby.

Canned milk is of two kinds; evaporated, which is unsweetened, and condensed, which is sweetened. *Evaporated milk* is whole milk from which part of the water has been removed, the milk then being canned and sterilized. The addition of water to evaporated milk restores it to the composition of whole milk in many respects, but it is still milk that has been heated. *Condensed milk* is evaporated milk to which cane sugar has been added to aid in its preservation. Since bacteria do not grow well in highly sweetened foods, it is not necessary to bring sweetened condensed milk to as high a temperature as the unsweetened product, to prevent subsequent bacterial decomposition. The high percentage of sugar in condensed milk quite obviously renders it unsuitable for continuous use as the sole article in a baby's dietary.

Milk powders or dried milks are prepared by rapidly evaporating the water from whole milk, skimmed milk or partly skimmed milk, leaving the solid constituents in the form of a light, white powder. Milk powder readily dissolves in water, forming a "reconstructed milk" which closely resembles the fresh milk from which it was prepared. But it must not be forgotten that reconstructed milk has been heated. Many doctors consider whole milk powder the most satisfactory form of preserved milk which is available for baby food. Should it be used, however, the importance of keeping it tightly covered and in a cold place must be recognized, for the presence of fat renders it likely to become rancid if not kept cold.

ARTICLES OF FOOD WHICH ARE SOMETIMES INCLUDED IN THE BABY'S DIETARY

Barley water, sometimes used to dilute whole milk, is made by mixing the barley flour to a smooth paste in cold water, adding boiling water and boiling for twenty minutes or cooking in a double boiler for an hour, straining and adding enough water to replace the amount lost in cooking. The proportions for different ages are as follows:

>Three months, ½ level tablespoonful barley flour to 16 oz. water.
>Six months, 1½ level tablespoonfuls barley flour to 12 oz. water.
>Nine months, 3 level tablespoonfuls barley flour to 10 oz. water.

Potato Water. One tablespoonful of thoroughly boiled potato is mashed into one pint of the water in which the potato was boiled and carefully strained.

Spinach. Spinach is carefully washed, steamed for half an hour and mashed through a fine sieve. It is sometimes started at the sixth month; one teaspoonful daily, gradually increased to one or two tablespoonfuls daily.

Orange Juice. The orange should be dipped in boiling water and wiped on a clean towel before being cut and squeezed, to avoid possible infection of juice. It is usually given to babies, sometimes as young as one month old, who take heated milk. It is carefully strained and started gradually by giving one teaspoonful in water once or twice daily between feedings and increasing to ½ or 1 ounce by the sixth month and 1½ to 2 ounces by the end of the first year.

Infusion of Orange Peel. This is sometimes used instead of orange juice, and is made by boiling one ounce of finely grated orange peel in two ounces of water, adding a little sugar to counteract the bitter taste and adding enough sterile water to bring it up to two ounces.

Tomato Juice. Canned tomato strained through a fine sieve, is sometimes given to a baby a few weeks old, starting with one teaspoonful and gradually increasing to four to six ounces daily.

Whey. One quart of whole milk heated to 98° F. or 100° F. and one half ounce of liquid rennet or one junket tablet stirred into it and allowed to stand half an hour or until firm and solid, is poured into a cheesecloth bag and allowed to drain for about an hour without being squeezed.

Protein Milk. The curd from one quart of milk, which remains after the whey is drained, as directed above, is mashed through cheesecloth in a fine wire sieve, with a potato-masher or bowl of a spoon and the curd washed through with one pint of water. A pint of buttermilk is added and the mixture boiled while being stirred constantly. This is sometimes given in diarrhea.

Beef Juice. One pound of thick round steak, slightly broiled, is cut into small pieces and the juice expressed with a meat press or a lemon squeezer, the amount varying from 2 to 3 ounces. It may be diluted with an equal amount of warm water, or slightly warmed by being placed in a cup standing in hot water, and salted to taste.

Broths. One pound of lean meat, all fat and gristle removed, is allowed to one pint of water. The meat is cut finely and put on in cold water, heated slowly and allowed to simmer for three or four hours, when water is added to replace what was lost in cooking. It is strained, the fat removed and slightly salted.

Oatmeal Water. Two level tablespoonfuls of oatmeal in a pint of boiling water is cooked in a double boiler for two hours, strained and enough boiling water to replace the amount lost in cooking.

BATHING AND DRESSING YOUR BABY

By the time you assume your baby's care he will probably be having his daily bath in a tub. It may be given under a spray, however, or the doctor may prefer to have him sponged. The sponge bath may be given in your lap or on a table covered with a pad, either method being satisfactory if the baby is kept warm and comfortable. But one inclines to the idea of having the baby bathed in the lap for he seems happier there; more comfortable and less frightened and we cannot be sure that these factors are unimportant to even a tiny baby.

The best time for the daily bath, during the first three or four months, is about an hour before the second feeding in the morning. After this age the full bath is sometimes given before the six o'clock feeding, in the evening, for a bath at this hour is soothing and restful and often helps toward giving the baby a good night.

Preparation for the bath should be made with its possible effects, both good and bad, in mind, for the baby may be helped or harmed according to the skill with which he is bathed. He must not be chilled during his bath, and fatigue and irritation must be avoided by giving it quickly and with the least possible handling and turning. These ends may be served by conveniently arranging all of the articles which will be needed, on a low table at the right hand side of your chair, before the baby is undressed.

There should be a pitcher of hot and one of cold water; a bath thermometer; two soft washcloths; soft towels; bath blankets; Castile, or some other mild soap; boracic acid solution; sterile cotton pledgets; large and small safety-pins, or large ones and a needle and thread if the band is to be sewed on; unscented talcum powder; sterile albolene or olive oil; soft hair brush and a complete outfit of clothing. The little garments should be arranged in the order in which they will be put on, the petticoat slipped inside the dress, and in cold weather, all hung before the fire or heater, to warm.

The temperature of the room should be about 72° F. and if it is possible to bathe the baby before an open fire or a heater, so much the better. In any case he must be protected from drafts and a sheet hung over the backs of two straight chairs will serve very well as a screen if no other is available.

The tub or basin should be about three-quarters full of water at 100° F. for the new baby; about 95° F. after the third month and gradually lowered to 85° F. or 90° F. for the baby a year old. The temperature of the water should not be guessed at, but tested with a thermometer, though in an emergency you may safely use water that feels comfortably warm to your elbow.

Lay a folded towel in the bottom of the tub, before beginning, as babies are often frightened by coming in contact with the hard surface.

It is a good plan to wear a waterproof apron, covered with one of flannel over which is laid a soft towel, until the bath is finished. The towel is then slipped out, leaving the dry, flannel apron to wrap about the baby. Wash your hands thoroughly with hot water and soap, before beginning; sit squarely, with your knees together, on a chair without arms; take the baby in your lap and undress him under a blanket. In order that the bath may be given deftly and quickly it is well to bathe the different parts in the same order every day, for practice makes perfect.

It is usually a routine to weigh the baby every morning, during the first two or three weeks and once or twice a week afterwards, though premature babies and those who are frail are sometimes weighed at longer intervals because of the inadvisability of disturbing them so often. The baby is undressed for his bath, wrapped in a blanket, and laid in the scoop or basket of a beam scale and a note made of the entire weight, for if he is placed in the scales without protection he is likely to be chilled and frightened. The weight of the blanket is ascertained separately and deducted from the total thus giving the baby's exact weight.

The eyes should be bathed first, with pledgets of sterile cotton dipped in warm boracic acid solution, each pledget being used but once. To prevent the solution from running from one eye into the other, the baby's head is turned slightly to one side and the lower eye wiped gently from the nose outward. The lids may then be separated by placing one thumb below the brow and lifting it slightly, and the eye flushed with a gentle stream by squeezing a freshly soaked pledget just above it. The head is turned to the other side and the eye on that side bathed in like manner.

The mouth is swabbed out *very gently* with boric-soaked cotton wrapped about the tip of the little finger, care being taken not to injure the delicate mucous lining. The nostrils are cleaned with little spirals of cotton dipped in mineral oil or olive oil.

The face is then washed with warm water, no soap, and patted dry. The scalp, neck and ears are washed with soap and water and thoroughly dried by patting and by wiping gently in the creases. The body should then be soaped with your hand, only one part being uncovered at a time in order to avoid chilling.

To place the baby in the tub, slip your left hand under his head in such a way that it will rest upon your wrist as your fingers spread out to support his shoulders. Your thumb naturally curves over and holds the upper part of the baby's arm without pulling or straining it. Grasp his ankles with the right hand and lower the little body into the water, feet first, as shown in Fig. 50. This gradual lowering of the baby into the water is worth while, for he is likely to be frightened if he is plunged in suddenly. If the baby's arm and shoulder are firmly held and supported by your left hand, it is an easy matter to steady his entire body and keep his head out of the water while giving the bath with your right hand, as in Fig. 51.

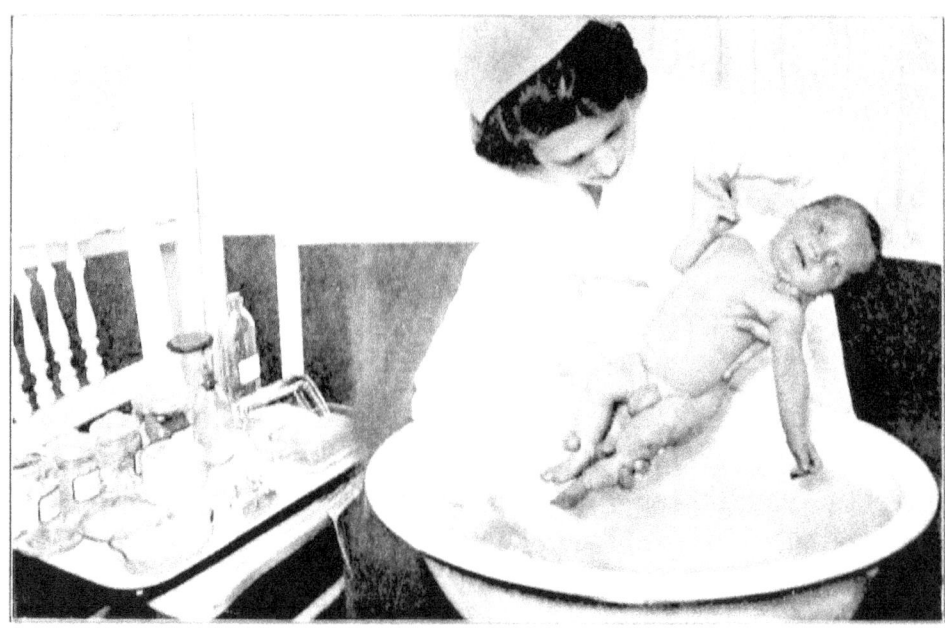

FIG. 50.—Method of holding baby and lowering him into his bath.

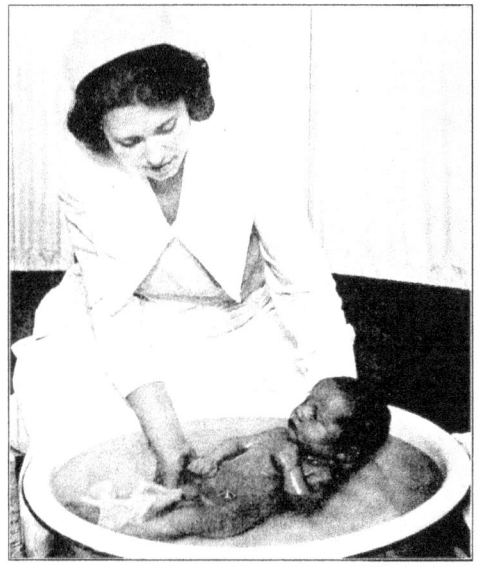

FIG. 51.—Method of comfortably supporting the baby's head above the water while giving his bath.

The new baby is not usually kept in the tub for more than two or three minutes, but when he is three or four months old he may stay in for five minutes and still longer as he grows older.

Hot water should never be poured into the tub after the baby has been placed in his bath but cold water is often added, for a three or four months old baby, or the warm bath followed by a quick sponge with cold water. The little body is quickly patted dry, afterwards, and rubbed briskly with the palm of the hand; the legs and arms stroked toward the body; the back from the neck downward and the chest and abdomen with a circular motion. Babies who react well to cold baths are benefited by them, but those who do not, may be harmed. Such "toughening" methods, to be beneficial, therefore, must be adjusted very carefully to the individual baby and should be employed only in accordance with the doctor's directions.

The **genitals** should be bathed and dried with care; inspected daily and any unusual appearance reported to the doctor. It is not uncommon for girl babies to have a slight bloody discharge from the vagina. Although this is unimportant and soon disappears, your doctor should be told of any discharge, however slight. The doctor often wishes to have the foreskin of boy babies retracted every morning at the time of the bath, by gently rubbing it back with gauze or cotton, taking pains that it is pulled forward to the original position after the part underneath has been thoroughly bathed with boracic acid solution. If retraction is impossible after several daily attempts, the baby is not infrequently circumcised.

The care of the baby's **teeth** is a part of the bath and should begin when the first tooth appears. It should be wiped front and back with a piece of gauze or cotton dipped in boracic acid or soda solution or some other weak alkaline wash, to neutralize the acid secretions of the mouth as these favor decay. After the baby has five or six teeth, the use of a very soft brush with tooth paste is often advised, the teeth being brushed with a circular motion or from the gums toward their edges. The teeth should be wiped, or brushed, morning and evening and after feedings. The reason for such close care of the temporary teeth is that they serve as a mold or brace to hold the jaws in proper shape for the permanent teeth which appear later. If the "milk" or first teeth decay or crumble away before the jaws are developed to the point when the permanent teeth appear, these second teeth are likely to be crowded, crooked and uneven.

After all of these details have been attended to and the entire body, including creases and folds, has been patted quite dry, it may be dusted with an unscented talcum powder, but this powdering must not be resorted to as an aid in drying the skin. In order to prevent chafing, the buttocks and thighs should be wiped clean with oil, or bathed with warm water, no soap, patted dry and powdered or oiled each time that the diaper is changed.

The **cord** has dropped off, in all probability, by the time you begin to bathe your baby, and the navel so well healed that you need do nothing to it, but you may be interested to know what painstaking care the nurse has given to this important detail of the baby's toilet. The form and method of cord dressings vary somewhat with different doctors but in practically all cases the dressings are sterile, to prevent infection, and porous in order that air may gain access to the cord and promote the drying process. The dressing itself may consist of dry, sterile gauze or gauze wet with alcohol wrapped about the cord, as shown in Fig. 52; or it may consist of squares of sterile gauze or muslin with holes in the centers to fit around the cord, and dusted with some such powder as boric acid, bismuth or salicylic acid and starch. The dressed cord is laid flat on the abdomen and directed upward to prevent its being wet with urine; a gauze sponge is placed over the dressing and the flannel binder applied, being sewed on or held in place with safety-pins, as shown in Fig. 53.

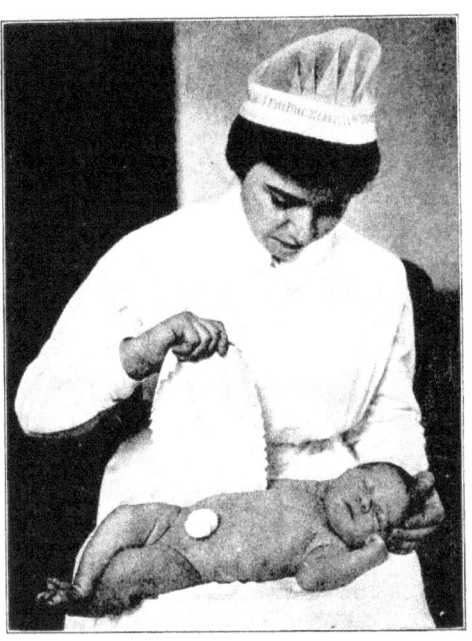

Fig. 52.—Cord dressed with dry sterile gauze. (From photograph taken at Johns Hopkins Hospital.)

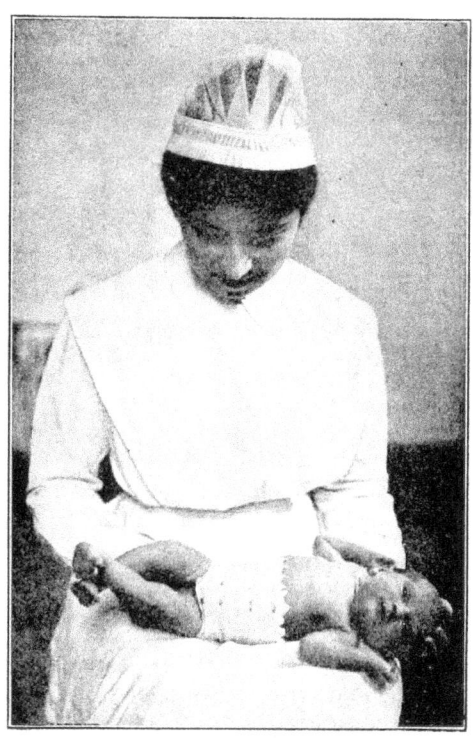

Fig. 53.—Straight flannel binder applied over cord dressing.

The band is put on firmly and with even pressure, but not tightly. It is a mistake to think that a tight band strengthens the baby's abdominal muscles, for it has quite the opposite tendency and in addition may give pain and even cause vomiting. The band is removed every morning at the time of the bath, or whenever it is soiled, but the cord dressing is not usually taken off unless it is soiled. When the cord finally drops off, the straight flannel binder is replaced by a knitted band with shoulder straps. This is usually worn for three or four months, particularly in cold weather, to provide a little extra warmth over the abdomen. Thin, delicate babies sometimes need this band for a year or more.

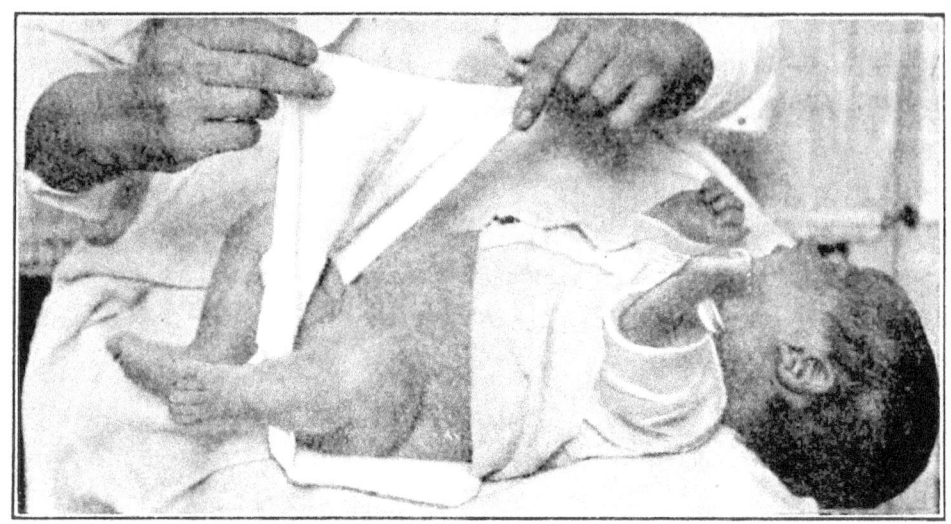

FIG. 54.—Putting on the diaper which has been folded straight through the middle.

After the band has been applied, the warmed shirt is put on and then the diaper. There are two methods of putting on the diaper.

One is to fold the square diagonally and bring the diagonal fold around the baby's waist. One of the lower corners is drawn up between the thighs, the two corners from the sides brought over this, straight across the waistline and not carried down between the thighs. The fourth corner is brought up over these and all are pinned securely with a safety-pin, while two other safety-pins hold the margins of the diaper together above the knees. The other method is to fold the diaper straight through the center, forming a rectangle twice as long as it is wide; to lay the baby on it lengthwise, draw the lower half up between his thighs as shown in Fig. 54, and pin it on each side at the waistline and above the knees. (See Fig. 55.)

In either case the diaper must be put on smoothly and care taken to avoid forming a thick pad between the thighs as this will tend to curve the bones of legs, which, as you know, are still soft. Squares of soft, absorbent material, which may be burned, when soiled, placed inside the diapers will greatly facilitate the laundry work.

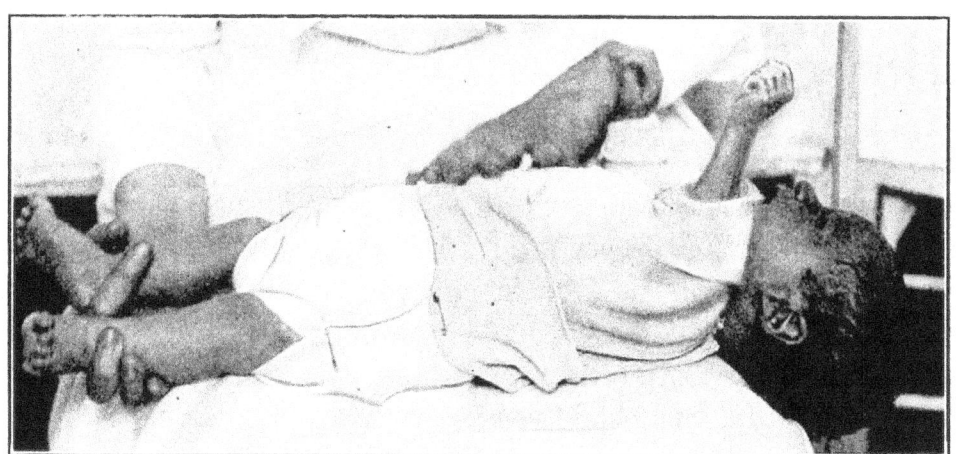

Fig. 55.—How the diaper in Fig. 54 looks after it has been put on.

The baby's diaper should be changed whenever it is wet or soiled, for in addition to making him restless and fretful for the time being, the skin about the thighs and buttocks will grow red and chafed if he is allowed to wear wet diapers. Wet diapers should not be dried and used again but washed with mild soap, boiled and whenever possible, dried in the open air and sunshine. All of this makes it apparent that the regular use of waterproof protectors is to be condemned since a baby so protected may wear a wet diaper for some time before it is discovered. Under special circumstances such as a drive, a short journey or visit the diaper may be covered by waterproof drawers but their habitual use will make the baby unhappy and uncomfortable and may even result in a serious condition of the skin.

Coming back to dressing the baby, after his bath, we find that after the band, shirt and diaper have been adjusted the petticoat and dress are put on with the fewest possible motions and the baby's hair brushed upward from his neck and back from the forehead. He should be wrapped in a small blanket, fed and laid quietly in his crib to sleep. If his hands and feet are cold a hot water bottle at 125° F. with a flannel cover, may be placed beside him.

When the baby is made ready for the night he may have a sponge bath or simply have his face and hands sponged with warm water, according to the wishes of the doctor. The clothing which the baby has worn during the day should be entirely replaced. The day and night clothing may be worn more than once, if clean and if aired between times, but it is better not to have the baby wear the same set of clothes for twenty-four hours at a stretch. In cold weather a tape is often run through the hem of the stockinette or flannel nightgown in order that it may be drawn up, bag fashion, to keep the baby's feet warm. During very warm weather the baby sleeps in a thin cotton slip.

YOUR BABY'S CLOTHES

Your baby's clothes were made long since, of course, but a word about their use is worth while as they may be very influential in promoting the baby's well-being. In order that his body may be kept at an even temperature the warmth of his clothing must always be adjusted to the needs of the moment. The general tendency is to dress the baby too warmly and the usual result is that he perspires; is listless, pale, and fretful; sleeps badly; is susceptible to colds and other infections and has poor recuperative powers. His digestion is likely to be deranged and he may have prickly heat. On the other hand, if the baby is not dressed warmly enough his hands and feet will be cold and his lips blue; he will cry from discomfort and the general result may be lowered vitality and disturbed digestion. If the baby's clothes are not comfortable, if they pull and drag or have tight bands, he will be fretful and restless, with disturbed sleep and upset digestion in consequence.

The little wardrobe will be entirely adequate, under ordinary conditions, if it consists of shirts, bands, diapers, flannel petticoats, dresses, nightgowns, flannel wrappers and sacques. As the petticoats and dresses are cut twenty-seven inches long, many doctors feel that they offer enough protection for the feet of the average baby to make stockings unnecessary until he is from four to six months old. The skirts are then shortened to ankle length and stockings added to the baby's attire. Other doctors think it wiser to put knitted socks or part wool stockings on the new baby, particularly if he is born during cold weather.

When the baby begins to creep, he should wear soft soled shoes, part wool stockings in cold weather and thin cotton or silk ones during the summer, and firm but flexible soled shoes as soon as he tries to stand alone or to walk.

During the first month or two the baby scarcely needs special clothing for outdoor wear as he may be wrapped in one of the flannel squares with a casing run in one corner to form a hood, or he may be placed on a square diagonally and the upper corner folded about his head and held under the chin with a safety-pin. The corners on the sides are folded about his shoulders, the lower one brought up over his feet and limbs and the additional blankets tucked in over all. But as the baby grows older and moves about in his carriage, he will need a cap and cloak or wrap with hood attached. In cold weather the cap should be knitted or wool lined and the cloak of soft woolen material or wool lined. In moderate weather the cap may be of one thickness of cotton or silk, or very light flannel, while on very warm days he will need no head covering at all.

To sum up: The baby's clothes should be simple in design, hang from the shoulders, fit smoothly but loosely and have no constricting bands; they should be of soft, light, porous material; their warmth always adjusted to the immediate temperature so that the baby will be protected from being either chilled or overheated. And his clothing must always be clean and dry.

AIRING YOUR BABY

An abundance of fresh air is one of the baby's greatest needs as it increases his resistance to disease and his recuperative powers, improves his appetite and aids digestion. In general, the more the baby is in the open air and the more fresh air he has while in the house, the better.

The two factors which must be considered in supplying the baby with fresh air are the condition and vigor of the baby himself and the immediate temperature and state of the weather. His age and the season of the year can be only partial guides because of the difference between individual babies of the same age and the variations in temperature, winds and moisture during any one season.

The air of the room which the baby occupies should be changing constantly in order that it may always be fresh, but the temperature should be equable and the baby protected from drafts. As the tendency here, as with the baby's clothes, is toward overheating, you will do well to remember that the young baby who lies covered up in his crib, may usually be kept in a colder room than is advisable for an older one who is creeping or walking about.

During cold weather the baby's bed should not be directly in front of an open window and he should be protected from direct currents of cold air by a sheet hung over the head and side of his crib.

Two or three times daily, while the baby is out of the room, the windows should be opened wide to air the room thoroughly, one of these airings being just before the baby is put to bed for the night.

The doctor's usual instructions concerning the temperature of the nursery are to keep it from 68° F. to 70° F. during the day and about 65° F. at night, during the first three months and lower it gradually to 64° F. during the day and about 55° F. at night as the baby grows older. It is customary to begin to open the nursery window at night when the baby is three or four months old, if he is well and the temperature is above freezing.

In planning to take the baby out of doors it is wiser, as a rule, to begin with the indoor airing when he is about a month old, except, of course, during the moderate or mild months of the year, when he is taken out at once. If the weather is cold, the baby may be protected with extra wraps and carried in the arms, into a room in which the windows are open and kept there for fifteen or twenty minutes. This indoor airing is increased by being gradually lengthened to two or three hours and by having the windows opened wider and wider. By the time he is two or three months old he is taken out of doors on clear, bright days, the best time being between ten and three o'clock, when the sun is high. If he is carried in the nurse's arms at first the warmth of her body serves as a protection and helps to accustom him to the out-of-door life, when he spends a good deal of his time out of doors in his carriage.

On windy, stormy days or when there is melting snow on the ground, the baby may be given his airing on a protected porch or in a room with the windows open. He is not usually taken out if the temperature is below freezing until the third or fourth month. After this time the average baby is taken out when the temperature is not lower than 20° F.

When the baby is dressed in his extra wraps he must be taken out of doors or the windows opened immediately, for otherwise he will become overheated and be in danger of chilling when taken into the colder air.

Warm hands and feet, a good color and the baby's tendency to sleep most of the time while out of doors are evidences of his being adequately clothed for his airing, while the reverse is true if he is not warm enough.

A robust baby who has been gradually accustomed to being out of doors during the day will usually be much benefited by sleeping out at night. But he must be protected from winds and his clothing so arranged that he cannot be chilled. Knitted or flannel sleeping garments or sleeping bags (See Fig. 20) are valuable and in addition, the blankets which cover the baby should be securely pinned to the mattress with safety-pins and tucked well under it at the sides and foot. The baby should wear a warm cap and the bed should be warmed before he is put into it. Or better still, he may be dressed for the night, put to bed in a warm room and the crib then moved out on the sleeping-porch.

An excellent device for protecting the baby's arms and chest, and keeping him generally well covered, is the poncho (Fig. 56) devised by Dr. Lucy Porter Sutton of Bellevue Hospital. The poncho is a rectangle made of flannel, outing flannel or an old blanket and cut large enough to tuck well under the head and sides of the mattress and extend below the baby's feet. The baby's head slips through an opening, which is almost a right-angled slit, equally distant from the sides of the poncho and about 20 inches from the top. The slit is firmly bound and provided with tapes to tie it together after the baby is put in. The poncho should be put on loosely enough to permit the baby to move about at will beneath it. After it is adjusted the bed is made up as usual with additional blankets.

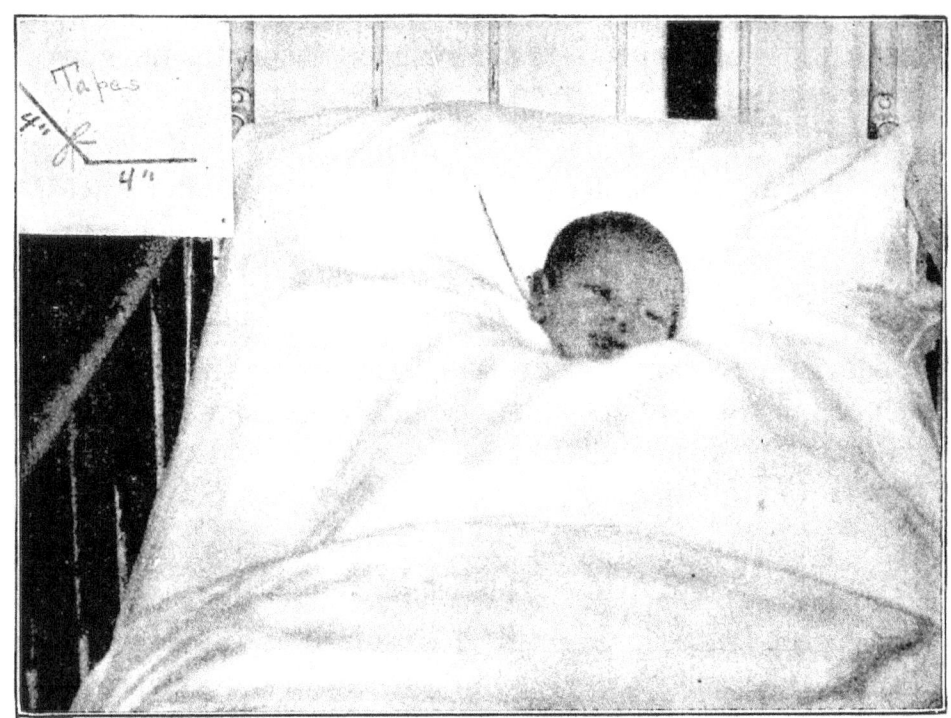

Fig. 56.—The "Sutton Poncho" which keeps even a restless baby well covered. The insert shows how to make the slit for his head to pass through. The regular bedding is turned back in this picture. (From a photograph taken at Bellevue Hospital.)

Under all conditions the baby's airings must be increased gradually, both as regards lowering the temperature and lengthening the time, and always adjusted to the vigor and reaction of the individual baby. He must be warm, but not too warm; he must be protected from wind and dust, and his eyes shielded from glare and from flickering light, such as may be caused by a tree in a light breeze.

EXERCISING YOUR BABY

Although the baby should not be handled unnecessarily nor tossed about and played with by friends and relatives, it is important that his muscular development be promoted by regular and carefully planned exercise. It is usually considered best for the baby to lie quiet and undisturbed in his crib most of the time during the first three or four weeks. Dr. Griffith begins the baby's exercise about that time by having the nurse or mother take him in her arms on a pillow and carry him about for a few moments several times daily. After a week or two of this form of exercise the baby is carried in the arms without a pillow but with his head and back carefully supported as the nurse is doing in Fig. 57. The position of the baby's body is changed by his being carried about in this way and the movement of the nurse or mother as she walks, causes a certain amount of motion of the baby's muscles which constitutes a gentle exercise. The baby should be carried first on one arm and then on the other in order that both sides of his body may be equally exercised.

This semi-passive form of exercise by means of being carried about is regarded by many doctors as almost indispensable to the baby's welfare. There is a possibility that lack of this form of "mothering" is one reason why babies in institutions sometimes fail to progress as they should. Certainly, it is inadvisable for the baby to be allowed to lie for very long in one position.

By the third or fourth month the baby sits up in his mother's arms, as she carries him about, and he may be placed on the outside of his crib coverings for a little while every day, to kick and struggle at will. His skirts should be rolled up under his arms, or removed entirely, to leave his legs quite free, care being taken that the room is warm and that he has on stockings.

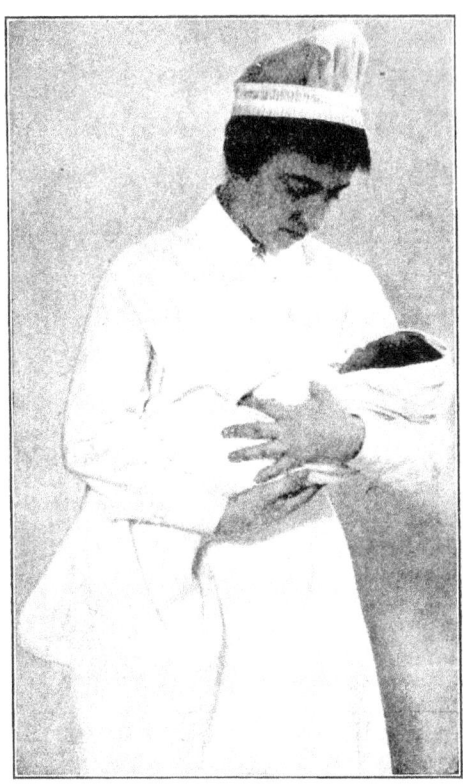

Fig. 57.—Method of carrying baby to support his head and back.

By about the sixth month he will usually begin to make an effort to creep, if turned over on his stomach and helped a little, and he may be propped up in the sitting position, in his crib, for a few moments every day. As he gives evidence of having enough energy to creep farther than the limits of his crib permit, he may be put into a creeping pen, or upon the floor under certain conditions. It must be remembered that the floor is likely to be cold, drafty and dusty. You should assure yourself, therefore, that the floor is warm and that all drafts are cut off, and then spread a clean sheet or quilt on the floor before the baby is put down to creep. When the sheet is taken up, be sure that it is folded with the upper surface inside in order that when it is again put down the baby will play on that side and not on the side that has been next the floor.

A creeping pen or cariole or some such provision is often more satisfactory than the floor, consisting as it does of a railed-in platform raised about six or eight inches from the floor.

The suggestions for exercise, like those for the baby's airing, must be very general since it should always be adjusted to the powers of the individual baby and directed by the doctor.

TRAINING YOUR BABY

Bowels. It is possible to train even a very young baby to have regular, daily bowel movements; and this training should be started when the baby is about a month old. At the same hour each day he may be laid on a padded table, or taken in your lap, a small basin being placed against or under the buttocks and a soap stick introduced an inch or two into the rectum and moved gently in and out. This slight irritation will usually result in the baby's emptying his bowels almost immediately. Another method is to hold the baby in a comfortable, reclining position, on a small chamber in your lap, as in Fig. 58 or with his back supported against your chest, and the desire to empty his bowels stimulated by using the soap stick as described. (A soap stick is simply a piece of soap about three inches long whittled down to about the size and shape of a lead pencil with a blunt point.)

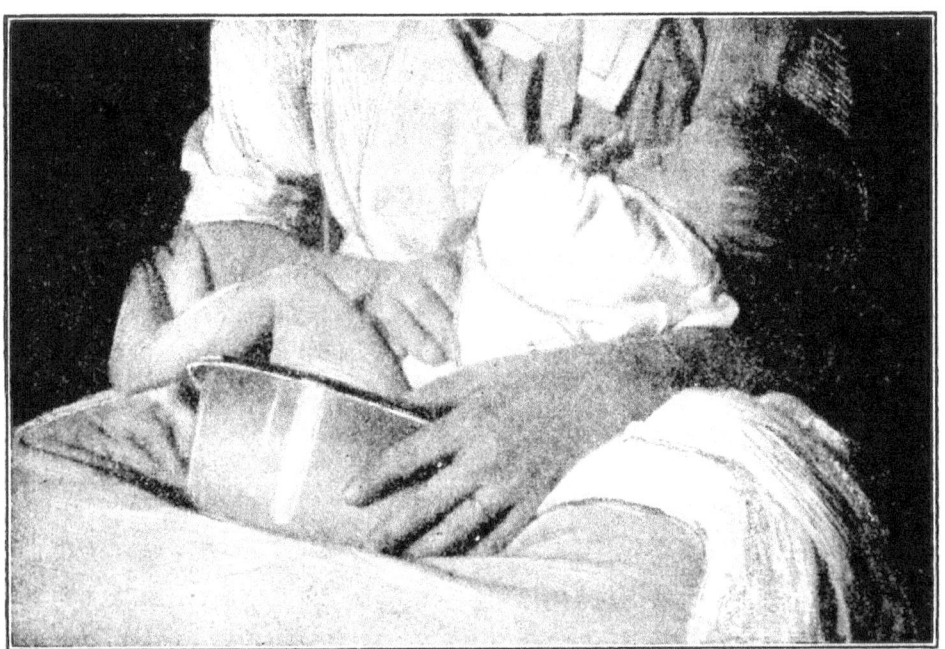

Fig. 58.—A comfortable position for the baby who is being trained to use a chamber.

It is of considerable importance that the position and method which are adopted, be employed at exactly the same time each day in order to establish a habit. If this is done and the baby is being properly fed, it will usually be found that before he is many months old, his bowels will move freely and regularly without the stimulation of the soap stick and only when he is resting on the small chamber or basin that he is accustomed to using. This establishment of a regular bowel movement not only simplifies the laundry work and the care of the baby but is of great moment to his health.

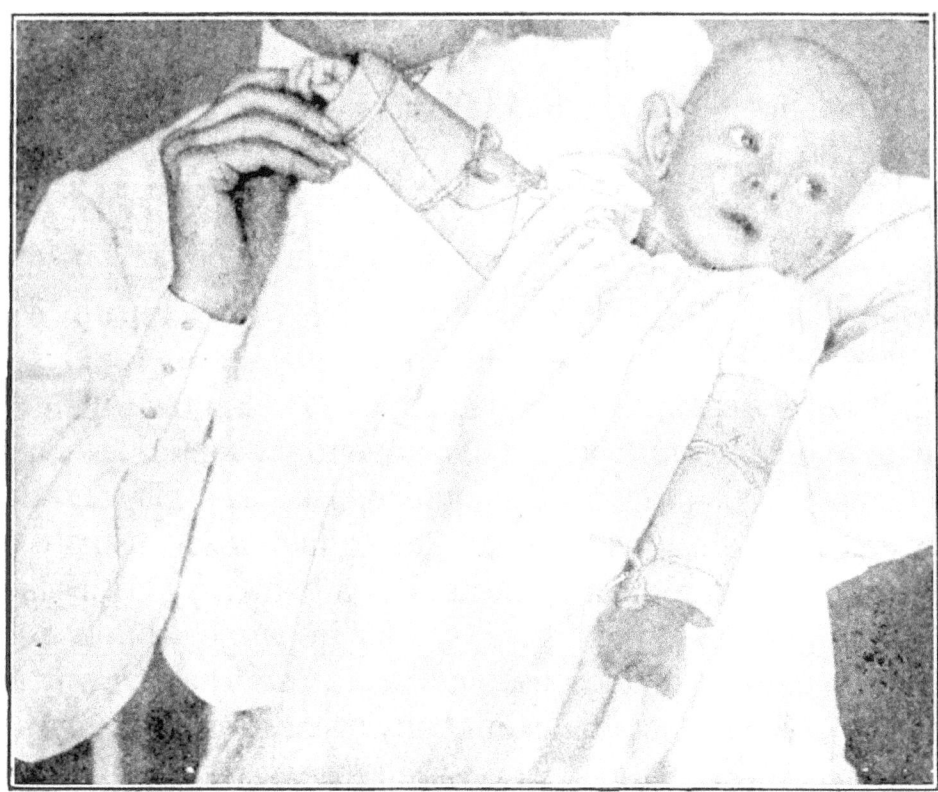

Fig. 59.—Stiff cuffs on the baby's elbows keep him from sucking his thumbs.

Thumb Sucking. It is scarcely necessary nowadays to tell a mother that her baby must not be allowed to suck on an empty bottle or a pacifier nor be permitted to suck his thumb. These habits are very dirty and help to spread disease. The baby may swallow air while practicing them, with colic as a result, and he may so deform the shape of his upper jaw that later in life, the upper and lower teeth will not meet as they should for satisfactory mastication; his front teeth may protrude in a disfiguring manner; and by narrowing and elongating the roof of his mouth, the structure of the air passages may be altered, with respiratory troubles and adenoids as a probable consequence. Thumb sucking may be prevented by the simple procedure of putting stiff cuffs on the baby's elbows, such as are shown in Fig. 59, and which make it impossible for him to reach his mouth with his thumb. These cuffs are easily made by covering pieces of cardboard with muslin and attaching tapes with which to tie them on the baby's arms. Another method is to put the baby's hands into celluloid or aluminum mitts made for this purpose, or little bags made of stiff, heavy material, which in turn are tied to his wrists; or his sleeves may be drawn down over his hands and sewed or pinned with safety-pins. It should be borne in mind that a baby sometimes sucks his thumb because he is hungry or thirsty and will give up the practice when his food is increased or when he is regularly given water to drink.

Ear pulling is not uncommon among young babies and, if allowed to continue, a long, misshapen ear may result. This may be prevented by using a thin close fitting cap which ties under the chin, or by using the same kind of elbow splints as for thumb sucking.

Crying. It is very easy to allow the baby to develop the crying habit but very difficult to break it up. The first step toward prevention is general good care, for a baby who is properly fed and exercised, kept dry and warm, but not too warm, and whose clothes are comfortable, will usually cry very little if wisely handled in other respects. But a baby may cry because he is hungry, thirsty, wet, cold, overheated, sick or in pain or simply because he wants to be taken up and entertained and has learned that the way to realize his wish is to cry. By examining the baby's condition and observing his habits, it is usually possible to discover the cause of his crying. Very often a drink of fairly warm water will quiet him, particularly at night. But unless he seems to have colic and stops crying because of the relief due to the upright position in your arms, you should hesitate to take the crying baby up and carry him about and hold him when it is discovered that this attention stops his crying.

Persistent crying should be reported to your doctor as it may be of some significance.

KEEPING YOUR BABY WELL IN SUMMER

Notice that I say *keeping him well*. There was a time when we looked upon the scourge, variously known as "summer complaint," "summer diarrhea" and "cholera infantum" as a seasonal visitation that was to be accepted with resignation. But happily those dark days are past, for though the condition itself is a complicated one, the one big factor in its causation was dirty milk—milk that was infected or spoiled or both—given to a baby whose forces were lowered by the heat.

It is perfectly clear, then, isn't it, that a baby is no more likely to be ill during the summer than at any other time, if he is given proper care, the kind of care that we have been going over in detail? Each of these details is important but just bear in mind that during warm weather it is particularly urgent to:

1. Feed the baby properly.
2. Keep him clean.
3. Keep him cool.
4. Keep him quiet.

The end and aim of these precautions is to prevent disturbance of the baby's digestion. As babies suffer from the heat more than adults do and are often excessively irritated and exhausted on warm days, these results of the heat are sometimes enough to upset his digestion unless he is safeguarded with greatest care.

It is much the same as with grown people, who often find that their digestions are upset solely by their being tired or excited.

The baby should have maternal nursing if possible, during the summer, for breast-fed babies fall victim to summer complaint much less frequently than de bottle babies. Quite evidently, then, you should regulate your own life with even more care than usual—for the baby's sake. He should be fed with absolute regularity, and as a rule, no matter what the nature of his food, it should be reduced one quarter to one third in amount when the days are very hot, and he should have an increased amount of cool, boiled water to drink. His weight may increase only slightly, or even stand still for a short time, as a result of his decreased food, but you need not worry about this if he keeps well, for the important thing is to avoid digestive disturbances. It is just the same as with grown people who are advised to eat less and lighter food than usual, while the weather is very warm, in order to keep well.

Cleanliness, as at other times, applies to the baby's food, clothing and surroundings. Many doctors think it safer to have all milk boiled during the summer, and of course expect scrupulous cleanliness in its preparation and administration.

The baby's soiled napkins should be placed immediately in a covered receptacle containing water, or a disinfecting solution and not left for even a moment where they may be reached by flies. They should be washed, boiled and dried in the open air and sunshine as promptly as possible.

The baby should be protected from flies and mosquitoes by screens in the windows and netting over his crib and carriage, both because these insects make him restless and irritable and because flies, particularly, are carriers of filth and disease—the kind of disease that kills so many babies during the summer. Accordingly, you should regard dies with deadly fear.

The baby should be kept away from dusty places and from cats and dogs. And since he will put his fingers into his mouth, in spite of you, it is a wise precaution to wash his hands several times a day.

The baby should be in the country, in the mountains or at the seashore, if possible during the warmest part of the summer at least, but if he is in town there is much that you can do to keep him cool and comfortable. His clothing at this season must be adjusted to his condition and the temperature of the moment just as it is in cold weather. A thin shirt, band, diaper and cotton slip will usually be enough for out-of-door wear, while in the house he may often dispense with the slip, and sometimes with everything but his diaper.

It is usually best to take the baby out of doors early in the morning and late in the afternoon, but to keep him indoors during the warmest part of the day, when it is likely to be cooler inside than out, particularly if the blinds are closed.

During excessively hot days, the baby will usually be more comfortable if he has two or three cool sponge baths, in addition to the soap and water bath, one of the sponges being given just before he is put to bed for the night. He should sleep on a firm mattress, preferably curled hair but never feathers, and in the coolest, best ventilated room available.

He must not be played with, held on hot laps nor subjected to the entertainment and attention which well-meaning but misguided mothers and friends are so eager to lavish on a hot, fretful baby.

Prickly Heat. Very often during warm weather a fine rash, known as "prickly heat" or heat rash, appears on the back of the baby's neck and spreads over his head, neck, chest and shoulders. As this rash is due to too warm clothing or to the hot weather or to both, less clothing and frequent baths will often give relief. If the baby is very uncomfortable he may he greatly soothed by being immersed, for two to four minutes in baths, at the temperature he is accustomed to, containing soda, bran or starch in the following proportions:

Soda Bath. Two tablespoonfuls of baking soda to one gallon of water.

Bran Bath. A cheesecloth bag about six inches square, partly filled with bran, is soaked and squeezed in the bath until the water is milky.

Starch Bath. About a cupful of cooked laundry starch to one gallon of water.

The baby should be placed in the tub as for his daily bath and his entire body submerged, as shown in Fig. 60, care being taken that his ears are above the surface of the water.

No soap should be used while the baby has prickly heat and after the bath he should be patted thoroughly dry and powdered with some such soothing powder as the following:

Powdered starch	one ounce
Oxid of zinc	one ounce
Boracic acid powder	60 grains

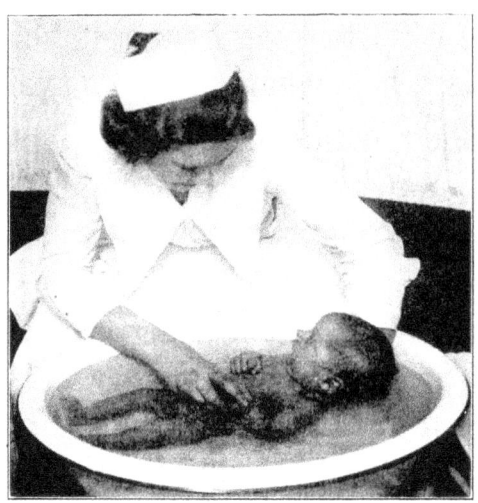

Fig. 60.—Method of holding the baby in the tub to keep all but his head covered, in giving a bran, starch, soda or mustard bath.

Diarrhea. If your baby has an increase in the number of his movements, or if they become watery in character, something is wrong. It may be only a mild disturbance or it may be the beginning of an attack of summer diarrhea, and as at first you cannot possibly tell which it is, you must not take it lightly. Notify your doctor at once, but if you are remotely situated or he is delayed in communicating with you, there are certain helpful things that you can do for the baby while waiting for the doctor. The first is to give an enema of half a pint of water, at 110° F., containing ½ teaspoonful of salt. (See Fig. 64, page 217, for method of giving enema.) If the baby seems to have only a slight diarrhea it may be enough to reduce his food one half, whether he is breast-fed or bottle-fed, and to give him an abundance of cool boiled water to drink. If he is bottle-fed it is a wise precaution to make up his formula with skimmed milk and leave out the sugar.

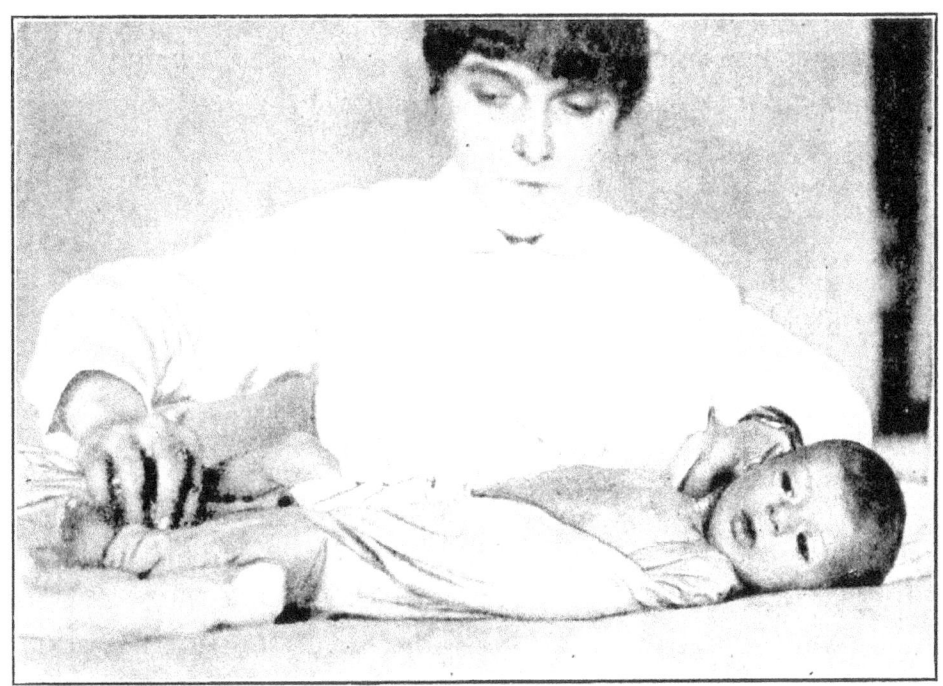

Fig. 61.—Putting the baby into a wet pack.

If the baby has frequent loose movements; seems feverish; vomits and cries as though he had pain, stop all food and give nothing by mouth but water, until the doctor comes.

If you care for your baby, yourself, through an attack of summer complaint you will find that the doctor's instructions are directed toward keeping the baby cool, clean and quiet, while he, himself, gives very careful attention to the question of feeding.

It is clear, then, that the baby should be lightly clad and kept quiet and undisturbed, in a cool shady place, out of doors as much as possible. During the warmest part of the day, however, he will often he better off in the house, in a room with the shutters closed. But while keeping the baby cool, you must bear in mind the harm that may be done by chilling him or exposing him to a cold draft or wind. The doctor may want him to have several baths daily, possibly tub baths, at a temperature of 100° F., or cool sponge baths. Packs, also, are given, for they not only cool the baby but quiet him as well, if he is restless. These packs may be cool (80° F.); tepid (100° F.) or hot (105° to 108° F.) according to the baby's needs.

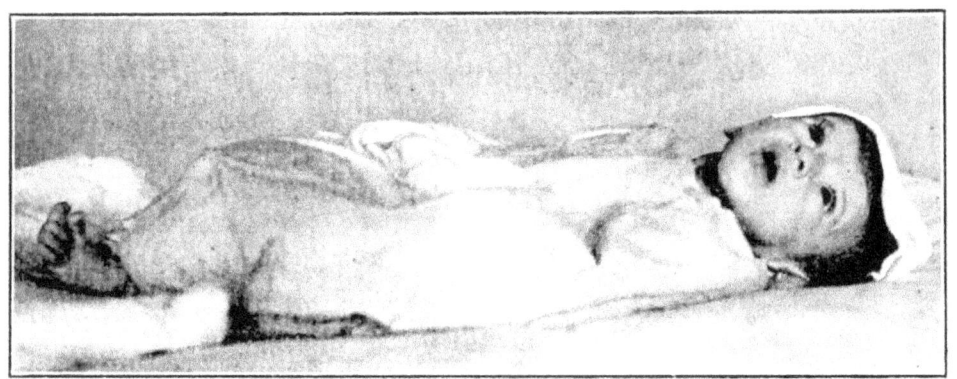

Fig. 62.—The baby in a wet pack with a hot water bag at his feet and cold compress on his head.

It is a simple matter to give a pack and you will enjoy doing it for you will actually see that your baby will grow quieter and more comfortable as you give it. Cover the bed with a rubber and sheet and bring to the bedside a basin containing a sheet wrung from water of the specified temperature; a basin containing ice and compresses for the baby's head and a flannel covered hot water bottle at 125° F., for his feet. The baby is laid on the upper half of the folded wet sheet, and an upper corner wrapped about each arm, as in Fig. 61, and the sides folded around his legs. The lower half is brought up between his feet and used to cover his entire body, being tucked around his shoulders. The hot water bottle is placed at his feet and an ice compress on his head, as in Fig. 62. If the sheets are wrung from warm or hot water, the baby is covered with a blanket after he is put into the pack.

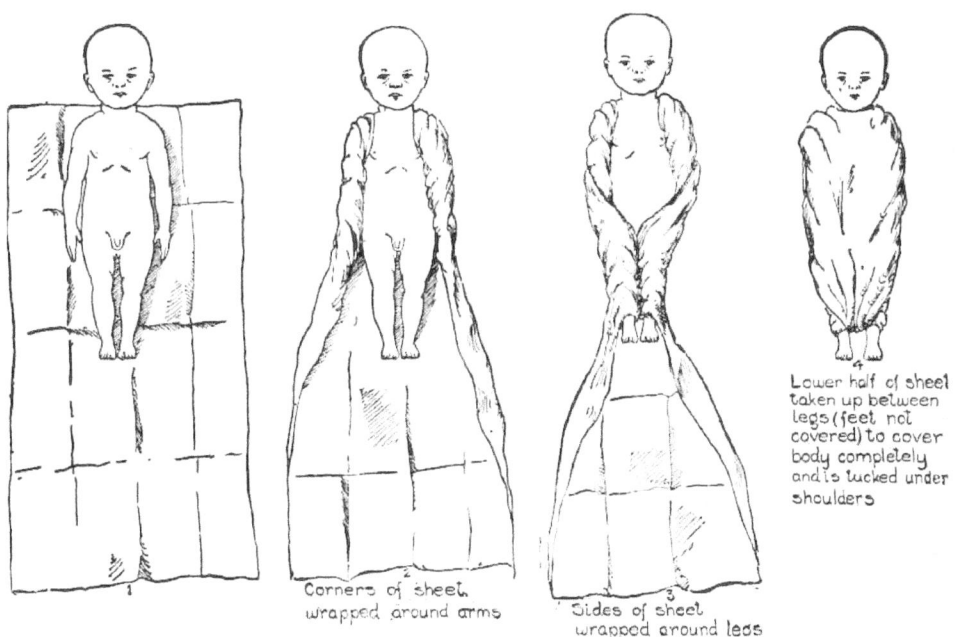

Fig. 63.—Diagrams shoving the successive steps in putting the baby in a pack.

Should your baby have summer complaint, remember that even a mild attack predisposes to another and you will have to be even more watchful and painstaking than ever, in your care of him. He will have to return to his customary diet very slowly, or he may not be able to take his usual amount of nourishment at all until the weather turns cool. Even though he gains no weight it is important to avoid taxing his digestion since it is already being threatened by the heat.

KEEPING YOUR BABY WELL IN WINTER

There are certain evils that beset the baby's way during the winter just as there are seasonal pitfalls in summer, but the truth is that if you care for yourself and him according to the suggestions that have been set down in the foregoing pages, you are doing practically everything necessary to make his way safe and comfortable. A baby who has proper food, plenty of fresh air, is kept clean and whose daily life is regular, is not likely to be ill during the winter or any other time.

The chief baby ills that come with the blustery weather are colds and the troubles that are likely to follow in their wake, such as bronchitis and pneumonia. Colds are infectious, you know, so keep the baby away from sneezy people and out of crowds and dusty places. If he should take cold in spite of you, send for the doctor at once. It may amount to nothing and clear up in a day or two, but if you let it run on, the dreaded bronchitis or pneumonia may result.

RELIEVING COLIC, CONSTIPATION AND CONVULSIONS

I have tried to impress upon you, at every step, that it is very unwise for you to delay in sending for the doctor when your baby seems ill, or to attempt to treat him according to your own ideas or those of your neighbors. But if the baby should begin to scream with colic or have a spasm, you would want to know what to do at the moment, and in case of constipation there are a few simple nursing procedures that you may employ to the baby's advantage.

Colic is always due to indigestion, whether the baby is breast-fed or bottle-fed, because of the food itself being wrong in some respect or because it is not properly given. The milk may contain too much of the material that forms the curd, or so much starch and sugar that fermentation takes place, the pain itself usually being due to undigested food or gas in the intestines. This condition may also result from the baby's being fed too rapidly or too frequently, or from his swallowing air while sucking on a pacifier or an empty bottle. Colic may be caused, too, by chilling the baby as this is likely to disturb his digestion.

Most babies have colic at some time during the first year, usually before the fifth month. The attacks may occur several times a day, after feeding, or they may not come on until the late afternoon or evening when the baby is tired. Colic is so common that most people are familiar with the symptoms: violent crying and a flushed drawn face; cold hands and feet; tightly clenched fists and a hard, swollen abdomen. As the pain is cramp-like, the baby stops crying every little while, and then suddenly begins again, drawing up his legs, doubling up his body and then straightening out with a jerk.

For immediate relief, you may give the baby a tablespoonful of hot water in which half a soda mint tablet has been dissolved, and an enema of half a pint of water, at 110° F., containing one half teaspoonful of salt, given through a small rubber tube introduced about six inches. This empties the lower bowel and enables the baby to expel a good deal of the gas that is troubling him so. Rub his abdomen with a little oil and apply a compress of several thicknesses of flannel, wrung from hot water, covering this with a larger piece of dry flannel, and change it every three or four minutes for a while. Place a flannel covered hot water bottle (at 125° F.) at his feet, cover him warmly, darken the room and he will almost certainly go to sleep. It is often a good plan to substitute barley water for one or two feedings, after an attack of colic, in order to give the disturbed digestive tract a rest.

Quite naturally, you must tell your doctor if your baby has colic for the cause may lie in the character of his food. But it may lie in some error on your part. Go over all the details of your share of the baby's care and see if you can discover anything to correct.

With breast-fed babies, prevention is often accomplished by the mother's nursing her baby more slowly, lengthening the intervals between nursings and by improving her own hygiene, particularly by relieving constipation and increasing her recreation and out-of-door exercise. Nursing mothers who lead sedentary lives and eat rich food very often have colicky babies as do those who are nervous, irritable and inclined to worry.

If the baby is bottle-fed he may be taking his food too fast because of an over-large hole in the nipple; he may not pause often enough during his meal or he may take in air as he nurses because the bottle is not properly held, as shown in Fig. 48.

In any event do not stop until you get at the cause of the trouble for though the colic itself may not necessarily be serious, a continuation of the cause may result in a run down condition or even in malnutrition.

Don't forget the importance of holding the baby upright over your shoulder after each feeding, to help him bring up gas, and of placing him immediately in his crib to be left quiet and undisturbed. And ask your doctor about drinking water. Very often the tendency toward colic is lessened by increasing the amount of cool boiled water given between meals.

Constipation is very common among babies and may be manifest by the stools being too small, too dry or too infrequent. It is more difficult to cope with than colic, though it, too, may have its origin solely in unsuitable food. In some cases, however, the constipation is due to absence of habit in emptying the bowels regularly; to weakness of the intestinal muscles; to long-continued undernourishment or to some such disease as rickets.

It becomes apparent that the prevention of this troublesome condition is accomplished largely by giving suitable food; constant fresh air; regularity in the daily routine and training the baby to empty his bowels at the same time every day.

When constipation is due to insufficient fat in the food, cod-liver oil is sometimes given, 15 to 30 drops three or four times a day; or a teaspoonful of olive oil two or three times a day. Maltose, malt soup, malted milk, milk of magnesia, mineral oil, oatmeal water and orange juice are all found among the remedies for constipation; while soap sticks, suppositories and enemas of oil or soapsuds sometimes have to be resorted to.

In giving an **enema** to relieve constipation, the baby should be protected from chilling, laid on a pillow and the bed-pan so placed that he will be comfortable and not inclined to move, and from half a cup to a cup of soapsuds, at 105° F., given with a small hard-rubber nozzle, as in Fig. 64. When warm olive oil is given at night (2 to 4 tablespoonfuls slowly through a small rubber tube introduced about six inches), it is very often retained until morning when the baby empties his bowels freely with little or no assistance.

Abdominal massage will often relieve constipation by strengthening the intestinal muscles, this in turn tending to make the bowels move. The abdomen should be rubbed with a firm but not hard, circular stroke, beginning in the right groin and working up to the margin of the ribs, across to the left side and down to the groin. This massage is often given for about ten minutes every day, preferably at night, but never just after feeding.

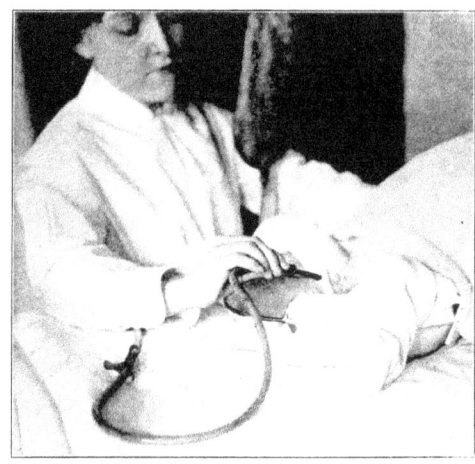

Fig. 64.—Giving the baby an enema. He is well protected, to prevent chilling, and lies comfortably on a pillow which reaches to the bed-pan, the latter being covered with a diaper where he rests upon it.

Constipation is sometimes entirely cured by nothing more than a suitable dietary; an abundance of drinking water; an out-of-door life; massage, and above all, the unceasing effort to establish a regular habit. These are all things which you, yourself, may do for the baby. The longer constipation persists, the harder it is to cure, so do all in your power to prevent it and if it develops, try to end it at once.

Convulsions are a symptom of several disorders of infancy and they may occur unexpectedly. Although at the moment, they are more distressing than serious, you should notify your doctor at once. If he cannot come promptly you may end the seizure by employing measures that will quiet and relax the struggling baby. The room should be darkened, kept absolutely quiet and the baby handled with the utmost gentleness. As a rule the most satisfactory course is to immerse the baby in water at 100° F. and keep him there for five or ten minutes, supporting his head above the level of the water as shown in Fig. 60. (See p. 209.) Have some member of the household place cloths, wrung from cold or iced water, on the baby's head and change them frequently. When removed from the bath, the baby should be wrapped in a blanket, kept very quiet and the cold applications to his head continued.

If the baby often has convulsions the doctor may instruct you to give him either a mustard bath or pack whenever he has an attack.

For a bath, one ounce, or six level tablespoonfuls of dry mustard is added to one gallon of water at 105° F. and the baby kept in it for about ten minutes, or until the skin is well reddened. He is then wrapped in a warm blanket and surrounded by hot water bottles, with cold compresses applied to his head. The mustard pack is given in the manner shown in Figs. 61 and 62, with a sheet wrung from mustard water which is possibly a little warmer and stronger than that for the bath, care being taken that the sheet is not cooled before it is wrapped about the baby. He is usually left in the pack for about ten minutes or until his skin is reddened, and then wrapped in warm blankets, with cold compresses to his head.

THE PREMATURE BABY

All of the precautions and gentleness which are necessary in the care of the normal baby, born at term, must be greatly increased in caring for the baby who is born prematurely. The premature baby is not only small, but in general is imperfectly developed, having slenderer powers than the full term baby, and at the same time much greater needs. His respiratory and digestive organs are less ready to act than those of the normal baby; his muscles and nerves are feeble; his heat-producing machinery is unstable and yet he loses an excessive amount of body heat.

Accordingly, the baby who has been deprived of those valuable last weeks of growth and development within the uterus, is small and limp; lies quietly most of the time; moves very feebly, if at all, and needs special care. To help him in maintaining a normal body temperature it is usually necessary for him to be oiled with warm olive oil and entirely wrapped in cotton batting or flannel or enveloped in a quilted garment, with hood attached, made of cheesecloth or flannel and cotton batting, such as is shown in Fig. 65. Diapers are often omitted in caring for very feeble babies, a pad of cotton, instead, being slipped under the buttocks, as this may be changed with less disturbance to the baby than a diaper.

A satisfactory bed may be devised from a basket or box with the bottom well padded with several inches of cotton, a small pillow or a soft blanket folded to the proper size, covered with rubber or oiled muslin and a cotton sheet. The sides of the basket may be lined with heavy quilted material, to shut out drafts and help to preserve an even temperature of the air immediately around the baby, or such a basket as is shown in Fig. 66 may be used. A flannel covered hot water bag at 110° F. may be placed beside the baby, or two, three or four glass bottles, each holding about a pint, containing water at 100° F. and securely stoppered, may be hung in the corners of the basket. A thermometer, also, should hang in the basket and the temperature kept between 80° F. and 90° F. The temperature varies less if the bottles are filled in rotation than if all are reheated at the same time.

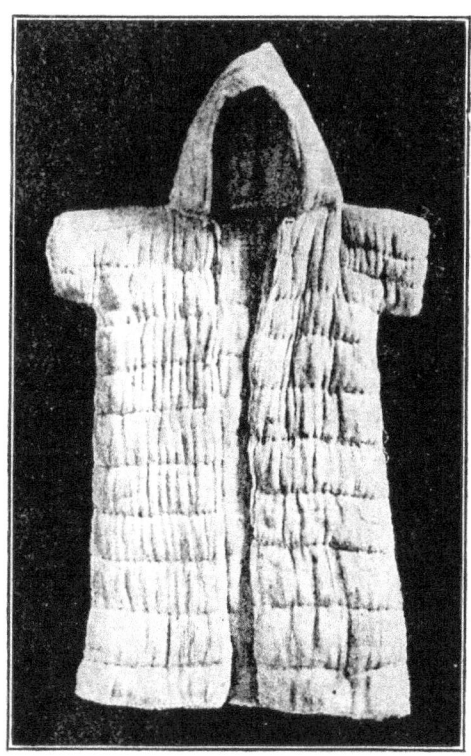

FIG. 65.—Quilted robe, with hood, for the premature baby. It may be made of flannel or cheesecloth with cotton batting for the padding.

The amount of heat needed around the baby is decided by taking his temperature (by rectum) at regular intervals; supplying more heat if the temperature is low and less if it is at or above normal. Some doctors have the temperature taken every four hours; others twice daily. As the baby grows able to maintain a temperature of 98° F. to 100° F., unassisted, the surrounding heat is gradually reduced and finally removed, and flannel clothing replaces the quilted robe.

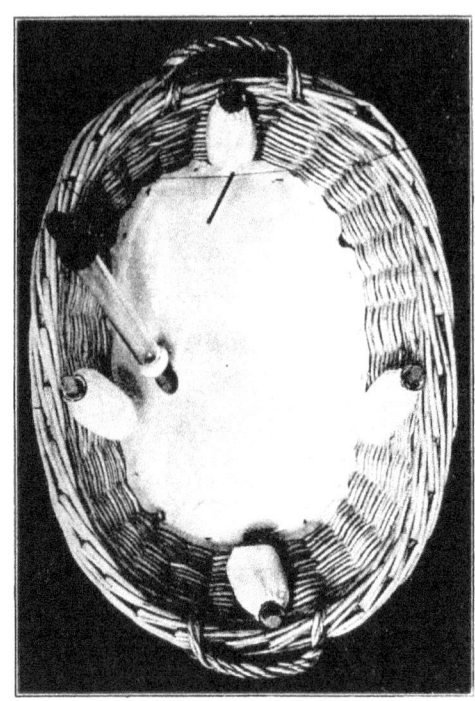

Fig. 66.—An improvised bed for the premature baby, consisting of a closely woven clothes basket with padded bottom and four flannel covered bottles of hot water, attached to the sides. The necessary thermometer and special feeder are shown in the basket. (By courtesy of Dr. Alan Brown, Hospital for Sick Children, Toronto.)

The basket in which the baby lies should be placed in a darkened, well ventilated room and should be carefully screened from drafts. As the baby needs moist air there should be a large, open vessel of water in the room.

Since the premature baby's lungs are not fully expanded, respirations are likely to be shallow and irregular, thus failing to supply the amount of oxygen which he needs. And as crying always causes deep breathing, it is a common practice to make the baby cry at regular intervals during the day.

In feeding the premature baby, breast milk is the most desirable food. In fact, many doctors feel that his life virtually depends upon it. If the baby is too feeble to nurse, the milk may be expressed from the mother's breast, being immediately covered and placed in the refrigerator unless used at once. Breast milk is sometimes used whole and sometimes diluted with sterile water and is often given from a medicine dropper or through a special feeder. Such a feeder consists of a glass tube with a small nipple on one end and a rubber bulb on the other, by means of which the milk may be gently expressed into the baby's mouth. (See Fig. 66.)

The premature baby's bath is of considerable importance. It almost always consists of sponging him with warm olive oil as he lies in his bed and with the least possible exposure and turning. It is given every day or every second or third day, according to his condition. The eyes are wiped with boric pledgets and the nostrils with spirals of cotton dipped in oil. The buttocks are wiped with an oil sponge each time the diaper is changed.

It must be borne in mind constantly that the premature baby is particularly susceptible to infection. He should be safeguarded by having everything that comes in contact with him scrupulously clean; being protected from drafts, chilling and dust, and allowing no one with a trace of a cold to come near him. The person who cares for him should wear a freshly laundered gown and protect her nose and mouth with a gauze mask while attending him.

TRAVELING WITH YOUR BABY

Babies should not travel; that is obvious. But if a journey is unavoidable, the attendant difficulties and disadvantages may be greatly lessened by making certain preparations. If the baby is bottle-fed, the preparations will depend upon the length of the journey and whether or not it will be possible to have freshly prepared feedings, for each twenty-four hours, put on the train from laboratories along the way. If this is not possible and the journey is not to take more than twenty-four hours, the entire quantity of food, ice-cold, may be carried in a thermos bottle. The requisite number of sterile nursing bottles may be taken or one bottle which is boiled before each feeding. Or the milk may be prepared as usual and the bottles packed in a portable refrigerator. Such a refrigerator may be bought or one may be improvised. The bottles are placed in a covered pail and packed solidly in crushed ice; this is placed in a second pail or a box with a diameter which is at least two inches larger than the inner pail and the space between the two packed firmly with sawdust. Several thicknesses of newspapers should be pressed down over the top and a tight cover fitted to the outer receptacle.

The sterile nipples may be taken in a sterile jar and a deep cup or kettle will be needed in which to warm the bottle before each feeding. It is usually possible to obtain water on the train which is hot enough for this, or cans of solid alcohol, a stand and a metal tray may be added to the traveling outfit. If fresh formulæ cannot be delivered to the train, daily, and the journey is to last more than twenty-four hours, one of the proprietary foods or a powdered milk will often prove to be a satisfactory solution to the problem of feeding the baby while traveling. The course to be followed, however, should be selected by your doctor.

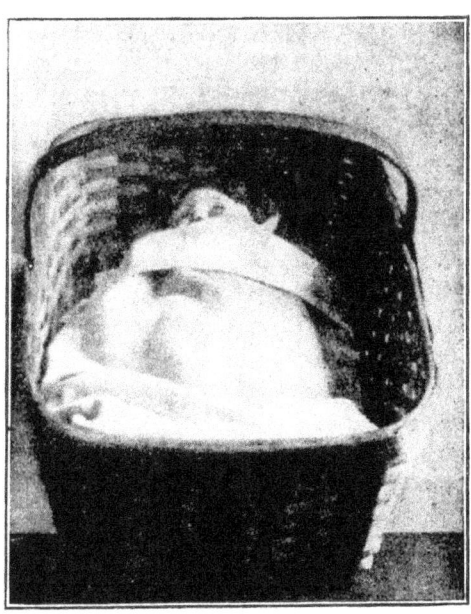

FIG. 67.—If traveling is unavoidable the baby will be comfortable and undisturbed in a basket converted into a bed. (By courtesy of the Maternity Centre Association.)

The baby will usually travel more comfortably and sleep better if he is carried in a basket. A large market basket with a handle or a small clothes basket will serve. It may be lined with a sheet or a blanket; have a small hair pillow or folded blanket in the bottom and be made up like a crib. (Fig. 67.) If this basket stands on the car seat during the day, and on the foot of your berth at night, the baby will be cleaner, quieter and less exposed to drafts than if carried in the arms.

As we look back over these pages of somewhat detailed description of the baby's care it is borne in upon us that the nursing of this unfailingly delightful and engaging little person has special adjustments and adaptations for different seasons and circumstances. But that on the whole the care of all babies, the year round, resolves itself into the observation of a few general principles, namely: proper feeding; fresh air, rest and quiet; regularity in the daily routine; cleanliness of food, clothing and surroundings; preservation of an even body temperature; consultation with the doctor at regular intervals and also whenever the baby seems ever so little ill.

If you are guided constantly by these general principles and apply them conscientiously, you may revel in the satisfying consciousness that you are keeping your pledge to your baby by giving him the best possible start on his life's journey.

CHAPTER XI
THE NUTRITION OF MOTHER AND BABY

Perhaps you are wondering, just a little, why I devote even a short chapter to the subject of nutrition when I have already given you suggestions about dietaries for yourself and your baby. I am doing so because this question of nutrition is one of such enormous importance in relation to the baby's future well-being that I want to give it special emphasis.

It is probably safe to say that the two most influential factors in creating and maintaining a satisfactory state of health are suitable nutrition and the prevention of infection. Although we shall concern ourselves solely with nutrition, in this chapter, it may be stated in passing that a state of good nutrition goes far toward protecting one from infection.

It will help to make the entire matter clearer to explain in the beginning that a state of good nutrition is not necessarily evidenced by one's being tall nor by being fat. But it is evidenced by normal size and development; sound teeth and bones; hair and skin of normal color and texture; blood of the normal composition; stable nerves; vigor both mental and physical; normally functioning organs; resistance to disease, and above all that indescribable condition which is summed up as a state of general well-being.

That this degree of nutritional stability is not as prevalent in this country as might be desired is disclosed by reports upon findings of the examining boards for army service, over a period of three years, and physical examinations of various groups of school children throughout the country. It was found in the first case, that about sixteen per cent. of the apparently normal young men who were inspected for military service, were undernourished in some degree, and according to Dr. Thomas W. Wood,

Professor of Physical Education, Columbia University, "Five million children in the United States are suffering from malnutrition." This army of undernourished children, which represents about one third of the children of the country, is on the broad highway to ill health, invalidism of various kinds and degrees, instability and inefficiency. They are certainly not developing into the clear-eyed, alert, buoyant individuals that go to make up good citizenry.

The tragic aspect of this state of undernourishment is that though a great deal can be done to nourish and build up the malnourished child or adult, a certain amount of damage that results from inadequate nourishment during the early, formative weeks and months cannot be entirely repaired later on in life.

As the baby grows and develops, certain substances are needed at the various stages of his progress, and if these are not supplied at these stages, there will always be some degree of inadequacy in the adult make up. It is much like the futility, when building a house, of using bricks without straw for the foundation instead of firm, durable rock, and then trying to make the structure substantial and secure later on by using good materials when building the upper stories.

The solid foundation and substantial beams and girders for men and women are put in during infancy and early childhood in the shape of good material that forms good nerves, muscles, bones, teeth and general physical stability. It is practically impossible to make up to the older child or adult for damage caused by failure to supply sufficient nourishment to the growing, developing, infant body.

> "The moving finger writes; and, having writ,
> Moves on; nor all thy piety nor wit
> Shall lure it back to cancel half a line,
> Nor all thy tears wash out a word of it."

We see all about us, the results of this form of neglect of babies, in the bow-legged, knock-kneed, undersized, misshapen, chicken-breasted adults and in those who are nervous and below par in endurance; are susceptible to colds and other infections and may be summed up as being "not strong."

The reasons for much of the undernourishment among people in this country to-day are to be found in certain widespread misconceptions of long standing as to what constitutes a state of good nutrition or malnutrition and the value and purposes of different foodstuffs. For malnutrition does not necessarily describe a simple condition due to an insufficient amount of food, but to any one of several complex conditions due to a lack in the food of one or more essential substances.

One may eat a large amount of food and even have a well-padded body and yet be seriously in need of certain food factors—in other words, be incompletely nourished in some particular.

That was possibly the first misconception—the belief that one simply needed enough food, and accordingly was well nourished if three large meals were eaten daily, irrespective of the composition of those meals. A step forward was taken when housewives and people generally accepted the fact that quantity alone was not enough to consider in providing food, but that the dietary should consist of balanced amounts of the five food materials: fats, carbohydrates, proteins, minerals and water, in order to build and maintain the body in a state of health.

But this, too, was found to be an error, in so far as it was only a part of the truth, for it was next ascertained that even provision for a suitable balance of the five food groups was not enough to nourish us, but that we must consider the heat-and-energy-producing properties of these component parts, as measured by the caloric unit, and that we must daily take in the requisite number of calories if we would keep our engines going.

It is now known that even this is not enough, for we may eat food in ample quantities, consisting of the properly balanced fats, proteins, carbohydrates, minerals and water, and it may daily yield the required number of calories, and still we may suffer from seriously faulty nutrition.

We find an explanation for this fact in the comparatively recent recognition of three substances, as yet not clearly understood, which are contained in a certain few articles of food, each one of which is essential to growth and normal health and well-being, though not necessarily concerned in the production of heat or energy. Various terms have been applied to these mysterious, but necessary substances, such as *vitamines, accessory food substances*, as applied to all, or fat-soluble A, water-soluble B and water-soluble C to designate them separately.

A surprisingly small amount of each of these substances is sufficient to meet the needs of an individual, but no one of these, even in this small amount, can be safely dispensed with, for if the diet is deficient, or lacking in one or more of them some form of nutritional disturbance will result. It may be severe enough to be diagnosed as a disease, or it may be only enough to keep the individual below a normal state of health.

When the disturbance is profound enough to produce a definite, recognizable condition, it is designated as a deficiency disease, of which there are three: scurvy, beri-beri and xerophthalmia. With these are sometimes included rickets and pellagra. The exact cause of the two latter disorders is not definitely known but both are associated with faulty nutrition. Poor hygienic conditions may enter into the causation of rickets, and infection may be a factor in the occurrence of pellagra, but neither disease appears in people who are suitably fed while both diseases may be produced by faulty diet and both may be cured with suitable food.

But probably of graver importance to the public welfare than the well defined nutritional disturbances, themselves, is the fact that between a state of good health and the level upon which a disease is recognizable is a long scale, along which is ranged an uncounted army of under-par, half-sick people. These are the ones who are tired, nervous, susceptible to infections, with feeble recuperative powers, and in general are more or less ineffective in the business of life.

It is this borderline state, or as Dr. Goldberger terms it, "the twilight zone," which cannot quite be called disease but is not health, that is serious to the masses, for diagnosed disease is given treatment, but nervousness, lack of energy and endurance, weakness and inefficiency are not treated; as a rule they are merely tolerated. The sufferers fail to reach their highest possible development and they fail to be of highest value to society.

This is the condition which can be so largely prevented by giving the baby a good nutritional foundation. This must be started during his prenatal existence, carried through the nursing period and then continued throughout the rest of his life.

It will mean much to the coming generation if the expectant and nursing mothers at large are able so to compose their diets that they will provide not only the requisite fats, proteins, carbohydrates, minerals and water and yield the necessary calories, but will contain, also, all three protective substances: fat-soluble A, water-soluble B and water-soluble C. It can be demonstrated that when these food factors are not present in the mother's diet, they will not appear in her milk, and accordingly will not be supplied to her baby.

That is the crux of the whole question. If your diet is faulty, your milk will be faulty in the same respect and your baby, being incompletely nourished, will start life with tissues that are lacking in those substances that are needed to make them sound and to promote health. That is what we have in mind when we say that the mother's milk must be satisfactory not alone in quantity but in quality as well, if the baby is to be well nourished.

In order to make quite clear how damaging are the results of diets which are deficient or lacking in protective substances we shall have a word about rickets and scurvy, the two diseases due to faulty diet, that are so serious for babies.

Rickets is a nutritional disturbance, common among babies who are fed solely or continuously on heated milk, either boiled or canned, and on proprietary food and sweetened condensed milk. Rickets may develop, also, among nursing babies whose mothers are on faulty diets.

The chief characteristics of the disease are arrested growth and softening of the bones, with dwarfism and deformities as a result. It is essentially a disease of infancy, occurring as a rule, between the fourth and eighteenth months but some of its unfavorable effects, such as bone deformities and poor resistance to disease, may persist throughout life. Although babies rarely die of rickets alone, it is one of the most serious of all health problems since it predisposes to such diseases as bronchitis, pneumonia, tuberculosis, measles and whooping cough and in general greatly weakens the powers of resistance and recuperation.

The common, early symptoms of rickets are irritability; restlessness, particularly at night; a tendency to have convulsions from very slight causes; digestive disturbances and profuse perspiration about the head. The baby may be fat, but is likely to be flabby and have a characteristically white, "pasty" color. The fontanelles are large and late in closing; the abdomen is large and the chest narrow; teething is usually delayed and the teeth may be soft, when they do come in, and decay early. But the most conspicuous effect of rickets is upon the bones which are soft, easily bent and broken and often misshapen. Their growth is likely to be retarded and the ends of the long bones may be enlarged, causing swollen wrists and ankles and the little lumps on the chest, so commonly called a "rickety rosary." The bones in the arms and legs may become curved as the baby lies or sits in his crib, making him either bow-legged or knock-kneed. Since the soft bones are easily bent their deformity is increased by the baby's walking or by the bunch which may be formed between the thighs by a large, improperly applied diaper. The spinal column may be curved, or too weak to permit the baby to sit straight or stand alone. The entire chest wall is often deformed, producing the familiar "chicken-breast" and so decreasing the size of the chest that the baby's breathing space is cut down. This is one reason why pneumonia is so serious with a baby who has, or has had rickets. The forehead is prominent and the whole head looks square and larger than normal, while the pelvic deformities in girl babies often give rise to very serious obstetrical complications later in life.

All of this, with the misery which it entails, is due to faulty nutrition.

The sovereign remedies in rickets are cod-liver oil and sunshine, in addition to general good care. But the treatment is a long, slow process, taking from three to fifteen months, and it is doubtful if the damage which the disease works can ever be repaired.

Rickets is more common during the cold months of the year, winter and spring, than during the milder summer and autumn seasons. A possible explanation for this lies in the higher value of the cows' food during the warm months when green things form the diets of animals. Since it is now recognized that milk is not a constant product, but that its properties vary with the food of the animals that produce it, cows' milk would be favorably influenced by their being put to pasture.

Similar evidence of such an influence is seen in the fact that although rickets is not seen among breast-fed babies whose mothers are on satisfactory diets, it may and does occur in breast-fed babies who are nourished by mothers who are, themselves, on dietaries which are poor in milk and fresh fruit and vegetables.

It is quite plain that a baby who is fed and cared for in accordance with the suggestions offered in the preceding chapters is not likely to develop rickets.

Infantile scurvy is seen among babies who are fed solely on milk that has been heated, boiled, pasteurized or canned, since the vitamine, in milk, that prevents scurvy is practically destroyed by heating or aging. That is one reason why it is dangerous to give stale milk to babies and why you should not use canned milk on your own responsibility. If the doctor orders it for your baby, he will know what to give in addition to the milk to keep the baby from having scurvy.

The disease develops slowly, the first symptoms appearing between the seventh and tenth months. Tenderness or pain in the legs is perhaps the most common symptom and may be detected first by the baby's crying when his diaper is changed or his stockings put on. And a baby who has been cheerful, playful and active will prefer to lie quietly and will cry whenever he is touched. He grows pale, listless and weak and fails to gain in weight or length. His large joints are likely to be swollen and tender; his swollen gums may bleed; his urine be diminished in amount and contain blood. But it is entirely possible for a baby to be in serious need of the vitamine that prevents scurvy and still not present these well defined symptoms of the disease. In such a case there may be stationary weight, fretfulness, a muddy complexion and perhaps tenderness of the bones.

Scurvy, of itself, does not often cause death among babies, but it is serious, nevertheless, for it makes the babies very susceptible to infection, particularly nasal diphtheria and "grip."

The disease may be either prevented or cured by giving orange juice, potato water, spinach or tomato juice to a baby whose diet consists of milk that has been heated and is therefore lacking in the vitamine that prevents scurvy.

Although scurvy is seldom seen in breast-fed babies it is believed that an infant who is nursing at the breast of a woman whose diet is lacking or deficient in fresh milk, oranges and leafy vegetables will suffer a certain degree of starvation and thus be sickly and susceptible to infection without actually having scurvy.

The significance to you, of this complicated and enormously important question of nutrition may be summed up as follows:

1. There are five recognized diseases resulting from faulty nutrition, which may be either prevented or cured by a diet which contains the protective substances, called vitamines, which are now regarded as essential to normal growth, development and well-being.

2. These essential substances are not necessarily provided in adequate amounts by a diet that is satisfactory in bulk or in its balance of fats, carbohydrates, proteins, salts and water or that yields the requisite

number of calories. The familiar diet of meat, potatoes, peas, beans, bread, pie and coffee is so far from providing complete nourishment that those who are limited to it are in a state of partial starvation.

3. Although the breast tissues are capable of converting into milk certain substances which they extract from the blood, they cannot create the protective substances which we have been considering. They can merely excrete these substances if they are contained in the mother's diet. The absence, or shortage of these food essentials in the mother's diet, and therefore in her milk, may result in rickets or other malnourished conditions in the baby, or in a degree of faulty nutrition which is not marked enough to be diagnosed, but enough to keep him frail; enough to give him the poor start that is so likely to put him, ultimately, in the class of those adults who are more or less unfit, though not actually ill.

4. The great protective foods are milk and leafy vegetables and any diet which is poor in these is incapable of nourishing satisfactorily.

By **milk** we mean fresh milk, first and foremost and also cream, butter, buttermilk, cream soups and sauces, custards, ice-cream and all dishes and beverages made of milk.

By **leafy vegetables** we mean lettuce, romaine, endive, cress, celery, cabbage, spinach, onions, string beans, asparagus, cauliflower, Brussels sprouts, artichokes, beet greens, dandelions, turnip tops and the like.

Other foods which are rich in protective substances are fresh fruit, egg-yolks and glandular organs, as liver and sweetbreads.

Nearly all of the common foods are deficient in some respect, but as the shortcomings of the various groups are different, we can arrange entirely satisfactory diets by combining foods which supplement each other's deficiencies. This explains to us why the meat-potato-peas-beans-bread-and-pie type of meals fail to supply adequate nourishment. These foods belong in the same general group and are deficient in about the same kind of food factors, thus tending to duplicate, rather than supplement each other.

If such a fare is enriched by the addition of the protective foods, milk and leafy vegetables, we have a well rounded diet in which the deficiencies of one group of foods are supplied by the properties of the other groups. In

fact, it is only by such a supplementing combination that an entirely satisfactory diet can be secured.

It is generally agreed that the two big problems of babyhood are proper nutrition and the prevention of infection, but nutrition is perhaps the greater problem, since any form or degree of malnutrition lessens the baby's powers to resist and to recover from infection. Whether breast-fed or bottle-fed, therefore, it is imperative that the baby be nourished in the complete sense of being given all of the food materials which are essential to normal growth, development and protection against disease.

If your baby is artificially fed on milk that has been heated you will understand why the doctor adds such protectives as cod-liver oil and orange juice, since the protective properties of milk are impaired by heating. If he is breast-fed, you will be able to supply to your baby the requisite nourishment and protective substances only if you yourself are adequately nourished and in good condition.

That is the point of this discussion; the fact that you must be on a satisfactory diet or you cannot satisfactorily nurse your baby. Satisfactory nursing means to give to your baby, from the beginning, through your milk, the materials necessary to build well and securely that temple, in the form of his body, which he will occupy throughout life; a structure so substantially built, from the foundation up through each successive stage, that it will be able to withstand the attacks of disease and weather the inevitable storm and stress of life, for perhaps even more than the allotted three score years and ten.

"The race marches forward on the feet of little children."